T0146347

Infectious Disease and National Security

Strategic Information Needs

Gary Cecchine, Melinda Moore

Prepared for the Office of the Secretary of Defense

NATIONAL DEFENSE RESEARCH INSTITUTE

The research described in this report was prepared for the Office of the Secretary of Defense (OSD). The research was conducted in the RAND National Defense Research Institute, a federally funded research and development center sponsored by the OSD, the Joint Staff, the Unified Combatant Commands, the Department of the Navy, the Marine Corps, the defense agencies, and the defense Intelligence Community under Contract DASW01-01-C-0004.

Library of Congress Cataloging-in-Publication Data

Cecchine, Gary.
  Infectious disease and national security: strategic information needs / Gary Cecchine, Melinda Moore.
    p. cm.
  "TR-405."
  Includes bibliographical references.
  ISBN-13: 978-0-8330-3989-7 (pbk. : alk. paper)
  1. Communicable diseases—United States. 2. Communicable diseases. 3. Epidemiology. 4. National security—United States. 5. United States—Defenses. I. Moore, Melinda. II. Title. III. Series: Technical report (Rand Corporation) ; TR-405.
  [DNLM: 1. Communicable Diseases—epidemiology—United States—Technical Report. 2. Communicable Disease Control—United States—Technical Report. 3. Security Measures—United States—Technical Report. WA 110 C387i 2006]

  RA643.5.C42 2006
  362.196'9—dc22
                                                                            2006024044

The RAND Corporation is a nonprofit research organization providing objective analysis and effective solutions that address the challenges facing the public and private sectors around the world. RAND's publications do not necessarily reflect the opinions of its research clients and sponsors.

RAND® is a registered trademark.

Published 2006 by the RAND Corporation
1776 Main Street, P.O. Box 2138, Santa Monica, CA 90407-2138
1200 South Hayes Street, Arlington, VA 22202-5050
4570 Fifth Avenue, Suite 600, Pittsburgh, PA 15213
RAND URL: http://www.rand.org/
To order RAND documents or to obtain additional information, contact
Distribution Services: Telephone: (310) 451-7002;
Fax: (310) 451-6915; Email: order@rand.org

Preface

The global community has suffered recently from newly emerged infectious diseases, including HIV/AIDS and severe acute respiratory syndrome, and from reemerging diseases once thought to be in decline. The world now faces the threat of a human influenza pandemic arising from the recently emerged avian influenza H5N1 virus. It has been increasingly recognized that infectious disease can have significant effects on U.S. and world security. Collection and analysis of information about the worldwide incidence of infectious disease is imperative for the United States to understand and respond to subsequent related threats. This study, conducted from July through October 2005, examines infectious diseases within the context of national security and assesses the need for and adequacy of information that will enable U.S. policymakers to prevent and respond to such threats.

This report should be of interest to those in U.S. federal and state agencies charged with collecting information about infectious disease and protecting the United States from its threat, the U.S. Congress, the world health community, and others who are interested in security and the threat of infectious disease.

This research was sponsored by the Advanced Systems and Concepts Office of the Defense Threat Reduction Agency and conducted within the Center for Military Health Policy Research and the International Security and Defense Policy Center of the RAND National Defense Research Institute, a federally funded research and development center sponsored by the Office of the Secretary of Defense, the Joint Staff, the Unified Combatant Commands, the Department of the Navy, the Marine Corps, the defense agencies, and the defense Intelligence Community.

For more information on the RAND International Security and Defense Policy Center, contact the Director, James Dobbins. He can be reached by email at James_Dobbins@rand.org; by phone at 310-393-0411, extension 5134; or by mail at the RAND Corporation, 1200 South Hayes Street, Arlington, VA 22202-5050.

Contents

Figures

Tables

Summary

The global community has suffered recently from newly emerged infectious diseases, including HIV/AIDS and severe acute respiratory syndrome (SARS), and from reemerging diseases once thought to be in decline. Additionally, it is increasingly recognized that infectious disease can pose a significant threat to U.S. and world security. To best understand and mitigate this threat, U.S. policymakers require adequate and timely information about the occurrence of infectious disease worldwide.

The Advanced Systems and Concepts Office of the Defense Threat Reduction Agency asked the RAND Corporation to examine infectious diseases within the context of national security and assess the need for and the adequacy of such information among U.S. policymakers. The primary objectives of this study were to assess the availability of information concerning global infectious disease threats and to determine the suitability and use of such information to support U.S. policymaking in preventing or otherwise responding to such threats. During the study, we conducted literature and document reviews, surveyed the current state of available information systems related to infectious disease, and interviewed 53 senior policymakers and staff from agencies across the federal government and from selected outside organizations. Our findings are summarized below.

Globalization Increases Both Risks and Opportunities

Approximately a quarter of all deaths in the world today are due to infectious diseases. In decades and centuries past, an outbreak of infectious disease was often limited to the locale in which it occurred. However, the pace of global travel, migration, and commerce has increased dramatically in recent decades, and that increase poses an increased global risk of disease. In the age of air travel, infectious disease agents can traverse the globe in less time than it takes for an infectious agent to incubate and cause symptoms in an infected person. As was seen with the rapid spread of SARS around the world, and into Canada in 2003, the risk of a new or reemerging infectious disease being introduced in the United States is perhaps higher now than ever. Certainly, the prospect of a pandemic caused by an avian influenza virus (H5N1 or another strain yet to emerge) has occupied both the U.S. media and policymakers in recent months; in fact, preparation for a pandemic influenza outbreak has recently become one of the President's top priorities. It is likely that such a pandemic would be enabled by globalization—frequent and unencumbered travel and trade.

The preparations for pandemic influenza being undertaken at the highest levels of the U.S. government highlight the link between infectious disease and national security. Obviously, the United States is concerned about infectious diseases crossing its borders, but the global toll of infectious disease also raises security concerns. Infectious disease can have significant effects that can lead to the destabilization of nations and regions through direct mortality and morbidity as well as staggering economic and social loss. Indeed, the U.S. State Department considers disease a potential war trigger.

While globalization has increased the risk and spread of infectious disease, there is no doubt that it has also benefited the world economically and culturally. Similarly, the same technologies that have enabled globalization also present opportunities to combat the threats it may pose, particularly in controlling infectious disease. These technologies notably include methods to collect and communicate information about infectious disease outbreaks more effectively and quickly than ever before. Faster worldwide notification of outbreaks can result in better and faster responses to contain them. Key questions, then, would address what types of infectious disease information are needed, and what information is currently available to U.S. policymakers.

The United States Has Responded to the Threat

The 1970s and 1980s saw complacency in the United States toward infectious diseases, in part due to a general perception that they no longer posed a significant risk. Infectious disease mortality declined in the United States during most of the 20th century. This trend was reversed in the 1980s and 1990s, yet it remained unclear whether infectious diseases were seriously considered in the national security strategy of the United States or other developed countries. The terrorist and bioterrorist attacks of September and October 2001 changed that posture. Since 2001, the United States has focused new attention on preparedness for detecting and responding to acts of bioterrorism. Legislation and executive policy documents have triggered a number of security-oriented initiatives directed at bioterrorism threats. It is clear that these initiatives, and their underlying infrastructures, are also useful for detecting and responding to naturally occurring outbreaks of infectious diseases. To policymakers involved in public health and bioterrorism preparedness, the relationship between infectious disease and national security is now clear, and it creates a need for timely and accurate information.

There Is Consensus About Information Needs

In recognizing that infectious disease and national security are linked, what kind of information do policymakers need to counter the disease threat? Does the United States employ a systematic approach to the collection of information for the early warning of infectious disease outbreaks originating outside its borders? Is adequate and timely information available?

We interviewed policymakers about their views on these questions and solicited their recommendations on how the assets of the U.S. government—across a broad range of sectors—

could best be harnessed to create a national information system, if warranted. While each sector has its own focus and responsibilities, the information needs of policymakers across sectors are characterized more by their similarities than by their differences. The policymakers and other stakeholders we interviewed expressed a strong desire for a centralized system that provides needed information to all stakeholders, and they described an ideal system as being (1) robust, drawing information from a wide range of sources and collecting information that is accurate and complete; (2) efficient, constituting a single, integrated source of timely information available to all stakeholders; (3) tailored to meet individual stakeholder needs and preferences; and (4) accessible, notwithstanding the need for protection of sensitive information.

Many Information Systems Currently Exist

To determine whether current systems might meet the expressed needs of policymakers, we compiled a database of Internet-based sources of information relevant to the public health aspects of infectious diseases, most notably disease surveillance. This database includes 234 sources from a wide range of organizational sponsors, including U.S. national and state governments, foreign national governments, and multilateral organizations. While they vary in their characteristics, these sources collectively provide abundant information. However, they do not meet all the needs of policymakers as outlined above. Most notably, there exists no single, integrated source of timely and accurate information.

The United States has recently funded an initiative that is intended to meet this need. The National Biosurveillance Integration System (NBIS) is based in the Department of Homeland Security (DHS) and is in the early stages of implementation; most policymakers we interviewed were unaware of its existence. While many of the 234 sources we assessed were focused narrowly in the way they collected information (e.g., reporting-based or Webcrawling) or in the type of information (e.g., animal or human data), NBIS is intended to be relatively expansive. NBIS is planned to combine data from multiple agencies—those with health, environmental, agricultural, and intelligence data—to provide all stakeholders with broad situational awareness that is expected to allow earlier detection of events and facilitate a coordinated response. Once fully operational, NBIS will insert these data into a common platform and combine them with environmental and intelligence data. DHS analysts are intended to work together with analysts from other federal agencies to process this information and present their analysis to the DHS Homeland Security Operations Center and an Interagency Incident Management Group.

Emerging Information Systems Require Evaluation

More and better information must be collected, integrated, and shared across government sectors that have, at best, a relatively short history of working together on shared priorities. It was suggested by some policymakers during this study that the United States needs a new centralized system for collecting, analyzing, and disseminating information about infectious diseases. Our main recommendation is for an integrated system that meets all the criteria and requirements described above. We recommend early formative evaluation of NBIS or any similar systems to ensure that they are designed to fulfill all critical requirements and are implemented as designed. During early implementation, it will be important to ascertain whether the systems are adequate or whether new or different strategies are needed to inform the broad range of policymakers responsible for addressing infectious disease security threats to the United States.

Acknowledgments

Many people gave generously of their time and expertise in support of this project. We thank John Zambrano, Arindam Dutta, and Martha I. Nelson of RAND for assisting in the search for online sources, and especially John for his work on the statistical analysis of the sources. David Hamon and Clete DiGiovanni of the Defense Threat Reduction Agency provided invaluable guidance from the inception of this project to its very end. We are indebted to our RAND colleagues Terri Tanielian, Michael A. Wermuth, and C. Ross Anthony for their careful and critical review of this work, and to Terri Tanielian and James Dobbins for their supportive and helpful oversight. Jennifer Gelman conducted a useful literature search for us, Monica Hertzman made thoughtful suggestions for the organization of the report, and Roshon Gibson helped us prepare the final manuscript. We are grateful for the comprehensive and thoughtful feedback on the final report from Ruth Berkelman of Emory University and Michael A. Stoto of RAND. Finally, the people who shared their insights with us in interviews are unfortunately too numerous to mention, but we thank them all.

Abbreviations

APEC	Asia-Pacific Economic Cooperation
ASEAN	Association of Southeast Asian Nations
BioSense RT	BioSense Real-Time
BKC	Biodefense Knowledge Center
CDC	Centers for Disease Control and Prevention
CISET	Committee on International Science, Engineering, and Technology
DHS	U.S. Department of Homeland Security
DoD	U.S. Department of Defense
EID	emerging infectious diseases
EINet	Emerging Infections Network
Epi-X	Epidemic Information Exchange
ESSENCE	Electronic Surveillance System for the Early Notification of Community-Based Epidemics
FAO	Food and Agriculture Organization of the United Nations
FBIS	Foreign Broadcast Information Service
G8	Group of Eight
GAO	U.S. Government Accountability Office, formerly U.S. General Accounting Office
GEIS	Global Emerging Infections System
GOARN	Global Outbreak Alert and Response Network
GPHIN	Global Public Health Intelligence Network
HHS	U.S. Department of Health and Human Services

HIV/AIDS	human immunodeficiency virus/acquired immune deficiency syndrome
HSPD	Homeland Security Presidential Directive
IHR	International Health Regulations
IOM	Institute of Medicine
LRN	Laboratory Response Network
NBACC	National Biodefense Analysis and Countermeasures Center
NBIS	National Biosurveillance Integration System
NGO	nongovernmental organization
NSPD	National Security Presidential Directive
OIE	Office International des Epizoöties (World Animal Health Organization)
PAHO	Pan American Health Organization
SARS	severe acute respiratory syndrome
UN	United Nations
USDA	U.S. Department of Agriculture
WHO	World Health Organization

CHAPTER ONE

Introduction

The emergence and spread of severe acute respiratory syndrome (SARS) in 2003 caused significant effects on the health, trade, and economies of a number of countries, particularly in Asia. Today, the world faces the potential threat of a human pandemic arising from avian influenza. While SARS did not cause significant mortality and morbidity within the United States, it served as yet another sobering lesson that emerging infectious diseases (EID) can have a significant effect on U.S. national security, with potential health, social, military, economic, and political effects. This lesson applies not only to newly emerging infectious diseases such as SARS, avian influenza H5N1, West Nile virus, and HIV/AIDS, but also to known diseases that have reemerged (such as tuberculosis and dengue fever), as well as emerging and reemerging animal (e.g., bovine spongiform encephalopathy ["mad cow disease"], foot-and-mouth disease) and plant (e.g., citrus canker) diseases.

The U.S. National Security Strategy of 2002 recognizes infectious diseases as a potential danger to the nation's security. However, it is not clear whether the links between infectious disease and national security are widely understood and how this new paradigm guides information collection and programming across government sectors. Current worldwide health information systems rely mostly on open and truthful reporting by governments. Such reporting does not always occur, either due to obfuscation (as appears to be partially the case with the SARS outbreak in China; see Chapter Three and Huang, 2003) or in part to the lack of a robust ability of some countries to detect and report human and animal disease within their own borders (e.g., HIV/AIDS in some African countries or avian influenza in some countries in southeast Asia).

Within the evolving new paradigm that links infectious disease to national security, what kind of information do government leaders need? Does the United States have a systematic approach to the collection of information for the early warning and tracking of infectious diseases originating outside U.S. borders? Is information collected by or available to the United States adequate for enabling a timely and effective response to protect national interests at home and abroad? These questions apply to a range of information collection sources that includes the more traditional health sector, the agriculture and foreign affairs sectors, and the intelligence community. How can the assets and approaches of these various sectors feed into coherent, integrated national information?

About This Study

Considering the need for good early warning information about infectious diseases that may affect U.S. national security or interests, the Advanced Systems and Concepts Office of the Defense Threat Reduction Agency asked the RAND Corporation to examine the evolving recognition of infectious disease as a national security threat and study how the United States collects, analyzes, and uses information about global infectious diseases. Data collection for this study was undertaken from July through October 2005, and analyses were completed in November 2005. The purpose of this study was to assess information priority needs concerning global infectious disease threats, and to determine the suitability of current information to support U.S. policy- and decisionmaking to prevent and respond to such threats. The research questions require careful consideration to help ensure that government leaders' information needs in this area are identified and met in the most efficient and effective manner possible.

The following questions guided this study:

- How has the emerging link between global infectious disease and U.S. national security been perceived and acted upon across government sectors?
- What types of information about global infectious diseases do U.S. policymakers need?
- How sufficient is the available information on global infectious diseases?

Study Methods

We employed several methods to address the central study questions. Those methods included literature and document reviews, interviews with relevant stakeholders, and a survey of online infectious disease information sources.

Literature Review

We undertook a literature review to provide background information on infectious disease threats and impacts, responses to date, the evolution of connections between infectious disease and national security, and key U.S. and global policies and initiatives. The literature and document reviews covered peer-reviewed literature, government reports, congressional testimony, and reports by nongovernmental organizations. Media reports were consulted for timely information about specific events. In the climate of near-continuous changes in global infectious disease information reporting and U.S. homeland security efforts of the past several years, every effort was made to review the most recent documents, especially guidance from the U.S. government and international organizations. We principally reviewed documents less than ten years old, and we did not include documents published after August 2005, except where specifically noted. The results of our literature review are presented primarily in Chapters Two and Three.

Interviews with Stakeholders

To examine all three of our research questions, we conducted interviews with policymakers and staff at various levels of government and with nongovernmental, academic, and international experts. We sought input from a broad range of potential stakeholders, mostly within the federal government. We targeted senior policymakers or their staff in all cabinet departments with a potential interest in global infectious diseases, as well as their relevant agencies. We also sought the views of relevant stakeholders outside the federal government, including representatives from a state health department, the association for U.S. state health officers, and the World Health Organization. We developed a discussion guide for our semi-structured interviews. Our discussions were more focused in a few instances when more specific information was required: for example, details about specific infectious disease information systems or new government initiatives. We conducted our interviews between July and October 2005. The results of the interviews are presented at the end of Chapter Three and in Chapter Four.

Survey of Online Sources

To supplement the findings from our interviews and in assessing the adequacy of currently available information related to global infectious disease, we conducted a systematic search for and analysis of Internet-based information sources. Our early literature review suggested no evidence for a comprehensive, consolidated source of information on global infectious diseases, and our pilot interviews with selected government officials suggested that this would be useful to them. Therefore, we compiled and assessed online sources that contained information relevant primarily to the public health aspects of infectious diseases, most notably disease surveillance information. Our findings are presented in Chapter Five.

How This Report Is Organized

Chapter Two provides background information to frame the challenges of infectious diseases and highlight recent U.S. and global responses. Chapter Three addresses our first research question related to perceptions about infectious disease and national security. It provides specific historical background on how infectious disease is related to concepts of security, highlights key U.S. security-oriented responses, and presents findings from our interviews concerning current stakeholder perceptions about the connection between infectious disease and national security. Chapter Four addresses our second research question related to information needs, summarizing findings from stakeholder interviews, and Chapter Five addresses the third research question related to the adequacy of current information, focusing on the survey of online infectious disease information sources worldwide. Chapter Six presents our synthesis, conclusions, and recommendations.

CHAPTER TWO

Background:
Challenges of and Responses to Infectious Disease Threats

Response to infectious disease threats is a long-standing priority of health agencies in the United States and around the world. The link between infectious disease and national security is a relatively new concept. Understanding the challenges of infectious disease threats from this perspective provides a background from which to address our research questions about information needs and the adequacy of currently available information. The first section in this chapter highlights the toll and challenges of infectious diseases; the second section describes U.S. and global responses in recent years.

Infectious Disease Threats

The Toll of Infectious Diseases

Approximately a quarter of all deaths in the world today are due to infectious diseases. HIV/AIDS, tuberculosis, malaria, pneumonia, and diarrheal diseases are the leading infectious disease causes of death and take a particularly large toll in developing countries (World Health Organization, 2004). In the United States, mortality due to infectious diseases decreased over the first eight decades of the 20th century and then increased between 1981 and 1995 (Armstrong, Conn, and Pinner, 1999). The average decline in infectious disease mortality rates accelerated from 2.8 percent per year from 1900 to 1937 to 8.2 percent per year between 1938 and 1952, then receded to an annual decline of 2.3 percent until 1980. Most experts attribute the declining mortality trends to improved water and sanitation and the introduction and widespread use of vaccines and antibiotics. From 1980 to 1992, the rate of deaths with an underlying infectious disease cause increased 58 percent (Pinner et al., 1996). Mortality increases in the more recent years were due to HIV/AIDS and, in the oldest age group, pneumonia and influenza.

The toll of infectious diseases over the past century can also be appreciated by comparing the leading causes of death at the beginning and end of the century (see Table 2.1). In 1900, four of the ten leading causes of death in this country were infectious diseases and collectively accounted for 31.9 percent of all deaths, including the top three (tuberculosis—11.3 percent of all deaths, pneumonia—10.2 percent, and diarrhea—8.1 percent) and the tenth (diphtheria—2.3 percent) (Cohen, 2000). In 2000, only pneumonia and influenza, which

Table 2.1
Leading Causes of Mortality, United States, 1900 and 2000

Rank	1900	2000
1	**Tuberculosis**	Heart disease
2	**Pneumonia**	Cancer
3	**Diarrhea**	Stroke
4	Heart disease	Chronic lower respiratory disease
5	Liver disease	Unintentional injuries
6	Injuries	Diabetes
7	Stroke	**Pneumonia/influenza**
8	Cancer	Alzheimer's disease
9	Bronchitis	Nephritis
10	**Diphtheria**	**Septicemia**

NOTE: Infectious diseases are listed in bold.

ranked seventh, 2.7 percent of all U.S. deaths, and a new infectious disease condition, septice-mia (ranked tenth, 1.3 percent), were among the ten leading causes of death (National Center for Health Statistics, 2000).[1]

Infectious Diseases in a Modernizing World

In comparison with the world before the end of the Cold War, borders are generally more open, and the pace of global travel, migration, and commerce has increased in recent decades. The effect of "globalization" on public health has been widely considered (for example, see Bettcher and Lee, 2002; Flanagan, Frost, and Kugler, 2001; Navarro, 1998; Roemer, 1998; and Yach and Bettcher, 1998a, 1998b). With globalization comes the benefits of increased commerce and closer international relationships, but globalization also presents new challenges and risks. One such challenge is that infectious diseases have followed a trend of increased global travel and spread. Just as infectious diseases are not confined to their nations of origin and have themselves become global in nature, appropriate responses to contain and control them have become a challenge to nations and require a global approach. This challenge has been addressed by the concept of global health, best described as "health threats and responses that, while inclusive of national governments, go beyond the action of nation-states" (Store, Welch, and Chen, 2003). While modern means of travel and migration have increased the threat of global disease spread by facilitating disease transmission among people and nations, modern times have also seen advances in the ability to recognize and treat infectious diseases.

Prior to the modern technologies that made rapid global travel possible, the geographic spread of infectious diseases was constrained by slower transportation: first, walking, then

---

[1]   It should also be noted that, while the number of deaths caused directly by infectious diseases is significant, infectious diseases also contribute to other causes of death, such as cancer.

travel by animal, then ships and trains. The historic role of travelers (particularly armies, explorers, and merchants) and animals (e.g., rats carrying plague) in the introduction and spread of disease is well documented (for examples, see Berlinguer, 1992, and Wilson, 1995b, 2003b). However, slower transportation and communications during those times also reduced the potential for early warning and response to outbreaks. As ever-faster means of travel have facilitated the spread of infectious disease, modern communications technologies have also presented the opportunity for faster worldwide notification of disease outbreaks. Faster notification, in turn, presents the opportunity for quicker response to control outbreaks. A critical challenge is to harness the opportunities of modern communications to address the modern challenges of infectious diseases.

Today, people can traverse the globe in less time than it takes for many infectious agents to incubate and produce symptoms. For example, SARS emerged in rural China, spreading to Hong Kong and, from there, to 30 countries on six continents within several months—and this was a disease whose transmission rate pales in comparison with that of influenza (Osterholm, 2005). (SARS is discussed further in Chapter Three.) Compounding the problem is the fact that many pathogens can be transmitted by asymptomatic or mildly symptomatic persons, including travelers, who may be unaware that they are carriers (Wilder-Smith et al., 2002). Also disturbing are reports that pathogens carrying resistance genes can be transmitted from person to person, and among asymptomatic carriers (O'Brien, 2002), increasing the spread and prevalence of antimicrobial resistance. Mary Wilson summarizes the problem this way: "Current attributes of the world's population—including size, density, mobility, vulnerability, and location—have increased the risks for many infectious diseases, despite the availability of an unprecedented array of tools to prevent, diagnose, treat, and track them" (Wilson, 2003a).

New infectious diseases are emerging at an average rate of one per year (Woolhouse and Dye, 2001), and at least 30 new or newly recognized diseases have emerged in the last three decades (CISET, 1995; World Health Organization, 1996). Modern-day infectious disease risks are not limited to human-to-human contact. Approximately three-fourths of infectious diseases that have emerged and reemerged in recent decades are zoonoses, i.e., diseases transmitted to humans from animals (U.S. General Accounting Office, 2000b). Examples include HIV, West Nile virus, SARS, monkeypox, and several of the hemorrhagic fever viruses. Such exposures are characteristic of human encroachment into new habitats. Zoonotic diseases also can be introduced into a human population via agricultural trade,[2] which is a critical element in many national economies worldwide.[3]

A crowded, interconnected, and mobile world has presented new opportunities for pathogens to exploit their inherent abilities to rapidly multiply, mutate, evolve drug resistance and increased virulence, and find new (human) hosts (Heymann, 2003; Rodier, Ryan, and

---

[2] The transmission of plant and animal diseases within and among countries poses significant risks to an affected country's economy and trade. Such agricultural diseases are beyond the scope of this report, which focuses more specifically on the threat of diseases directly relevant to humans, including zoonotic diseases.

[3] Significantly for the United States, due to its high volume of international trade, zoonoses may also be introduced by the inadvertent introduction of animals. For example, as of this writing, the United States imports approximately 9 million sea shipping containers per year (U.S. Customs and Border Protection, undated). These containers may include animals or other biologics, either intentionally via trade or unintentionally as "stowaways." The 2003 cases of monkeypox arising

Heymann, 2000). Rapid and unplanned urbanization, particularly in developing countries, poses yet another set of risks for infectious disease transmission. Specific risk factors include poor sanitation, crowding, and sharing resources such as food and water (Moore, Gould, and Keary, 2003). As Heymann (2003) points out with numerous examples, the modernization of global trade and travel has resulted in the unprecedented emergence of new diseases, the reemergence of known diseases, and growing antimicrobial resistance.

Near-Term Infectious Disease Threat: Avian Influenza

As of this writing, the H5N1 strain of influenza (avian influenza) has raced through bird populations in Asia and into eastern Europe, and has been documented to have jumped to humans in some instances, with 204 officially reported cases (most of whom had direct contact with infected birds) and 113 deaths in nine countries since 2003. It is widely feared that this virus will adapt sufficiently to permit efficient human-to-human transmission, either through mutations or through reassortment with a human influenza virus, resulting in a novel strain that spreads easily among people. This could trigger a human influenza pandemic that could potentially kill millions of people worldwide (estimates range from 2–7.4 million to 71 million), proportionally rivaling the Spanish influenza pandemic of 1918–1919 (McKibben and Sidorenko, 2006).[4] Estimates vary on the worldwide death toll of the 1918–1919 pandemic, but most estimates range from 20 to 50 million (Lederberg, 1997; Mills, Robins, and Lipsitch, 2004; Trampuz et al., 2004) or 50 to 100 million (Johnson and Mueller, 2002; Oxford et al., 2005) deaths. While various experts offer a wide range of projections, the Centers for Disease Control and Prevention (CDC) predicted that a "medium-level epidemic" could kill up to 207,000 Americans and sicken about a third of the U.S. population (Crosse, 2005), and a larger epidemic of avian influenza could be even more devastating, perhaps resulting in 16 million U.S. deaths (Garrett, 2005). The *HHS Pandemic Influenza Plan*, released in November 2005, includes planning assumptions that 30 percent of the U.S. population will become sick and 209,000 to 1.9 million will die in moderate and severe pandemic scenarios, respectively (U.S. Department of Health and Human Services, 2005; see also White House, 2005).

In September 2005, President George W. Bush established an "International Partnership on Avian and Pandemic Influenza" to coordinate global response strategies. Senate Majority Leader Bill Frist (who is a physician) opined that the United States is "dangerously unprepared to defend" against avian influenza, calling for an "all-out effort to defend against the threat of human-made and naturally occurring infectious diseases" (Frist, 2005). Interviews conducted during this study indicated that pandemic influenza response was among the President's top five national priorities as early as summer 2005. However, multiple interviewees in this study

---

from the importation of wild rodent pets from Ghana into the United States is an example of the former, and the historical spread of bubonic plague by way of rats is an example of the latter. This annual volume reflects an increase of more than 3 million containers since 2001 (Fields, 2002). Of particular concern because of their small size and ubiquity are rats and arthropod vectors of diseases that are transported inadvertently (Lounibos, 2002) and may successfully establish populations in new locations (Moore and Mitchell, 1997), sometimes without natural predators or other environmental controls.

[4] See also World Health Organization (2005b).

also informed us that there is some evidence that nations are reluctant to report outbreaks of avian influenza among birds or humans, fearing significant economic costs related to preventive culling of bird flocks and reduced travel and trade.

While globalization has changed the world in ways that can foster the spread of infectious disease, it has also changed traditional concepts of security. The remainder of this chapter provides background information about U.S. and global responses to the threat of infectious diseases.

Responses to Threats from Infectious Disease

Interest in infectious disease surveillance and response increased in the United States and, subsequently, in the broader world community during the 1990s, probably due to a combination of factors. First, at least in the United States, the emergence and resurgence of infectious diseases since 1980 erased the attitude that the war against infectious disease had been won; second, policymakers appreciated more fully the effect of globalization on the spread of infectious disease; and third, they recognized the increasing and profound global effect of HIV/AIDS.

U.S. Response

The 1970s and 1980s saw complacency in the United States toward infectious diseases, in part due to a general perception that infectious diseases no longer posed a significant risk. Smallpox was eradicated (the last naturally occurring case was in 1977), and other infectious diseases, such as tuberculosis, seemed to be controlled. Indeed, U.S. public health literature is rife with descriptions of such complacency. William Stewart, U.S. Surgeon General from 1965 to 1969, is widely quoted as having "closed the book on infectious diseases" in 1969 and redirecting public health priorities toward noncommunicable chronic diseases (Stewart, 1967; Lederberg, Shope, and Oaks, 1992). (Of note, the U.S. Public Health Service historian was unable to confirm that Dr. Stewart ever made such a statement in the congressional record, as it is often cited.) State and federal spending on infectious disease surveillance and control declined throughout the 1980s. However, during this same period—the 1970s and 1980s—new infectious diseases began to appear: Legionnaire's disease, Ebola, E. coli H7:0157, HIV/AIDS, and others, and the prevalence of older diseases, including tuberculosis, malaria, and dengue fever, increased.

By the early 1990s, infectious diseases began once again to attract attention on the public policy agenda:

- In 1992, the Institute of Medicine (IOM) issued its landmark report, *Emerging Infections: Microbial Threats to Health in the United States*, triggering heightened awareness of the resurgence of infectious diseases and the need for adequate public health and medical infrastructures to control them (Lederberg, Shope, and Oaks, 1992).
- In 1994, the CDC issued its first comprehensive national strategy on emerging infectious diseases (CDC, 1994).

- In 1995, a U.S. National Science and Technology Council working group issued a comparable strategy with a global reach, based on the evolving view that infectious diseases pose challenges to foreign policy and could constitute a threat to national security (CISET, 1995).
- In 1996, President Clinton issued a Presidential Decision Directive (White House, 1996a) to implement elements of that strategy. The directive included a policy goal of "establish[ing] a global infectious disease surveillance and response system, based on regional hubs and linked by modern communications." On the same day, Vice President Gore declared that "emerging infectious diseases present one of the most significant health and security challenges facing the global community" (White House, 1996b).
- In 1997, the IOM published another landmark report, *America's Vital Interest in Global Health* (Institute of Medicine, 1997), to "sell" the importance of global health and infectious diseases to the American public.
- In 1998, the CDC updated its national EID strategy (CDC, 1998).

As more policy attention began to be paid to the potential security threat of global infectious disease, the U.S. National Intelligence Council prepared a report on the future threat of infectious diseases in response to "a growing concern by senior U.S. leaders" (U.S. National Intelligence Council, 2000). The report examined alternative future scenarios that looked forward 20 years. It concluded that the most likely scenario is one in which the infectious disease threat worsens during the first half of that time frame but "decreases fitfully" thereafter due to improved prevention, control, drugs and vaccines, and socioeconomic improvements. This estimate, prepared before the emergence of SARS and the more recent spread of avian influenza, concluded this scenario to be the most likely, barring the appearance of a deadly and highly infectious new disease. The report stated that

- "New and reemerging infectious diseases will . . . complicate U.S. and global security over the next 20 years. These diseases will endanger U.S. citizens at home and abroad, threaten armed forces deployed overseas, and exacerbate social and political instability in key countries and regions in which the United States has significant interests" (p. 5).
- "The relationship between disease and political instability is indirect but real" (p. 10).
- "The severe social and economic impact of infectious diseases is likely to intensify the struggle for political power to control state resources" (p. 10).
- The spread of HIV/AIDS in Africa, together with other factors of instability, could jeopardize U.S. national security and national interests (p. 54).

Global Response
Complacency at the global level during the 1970s mirrored that in the United States. The landmark 1978 WHO "Health for All 2000" strategy, which predicted that even poor nations would see improvements in health before the millennium, epitomized the optimism that global infectious diseases could be managed and would not present a significant future threat (see

World Health Organization, 1978). However, by the 1990s, multilateral organizations also began to recognize and respond to the growing global threat of infectious diseases:

- In May 1995, the World Health Organization (WHO) passed a resolution urging member states to strengthen surveillance and reporting of emerging infectious diseases (World Health Assembly, 1995).
- In January 2000, by U.S. example, the United Nations Security Council considered a health issue for the first time, concluding that HIV/AIDS presented a threat to economic development, global security, and the viability of states (United Nations Security Council, 2000).
- Also in 2000, the Group of Eight (G8), at its meeting in Okinawa, Japan, acknowledged the need for an international mechanism to fund the surveillance and control of infectious diseases.
- In May 2001, U.S. President Bush and the UN Secretary-General called for the establishment of an international relief fund directed at three killer diseases. The Global Fund to Fight AIDS, Tuberculosis and Malaria is a federation registered under Swiss law and represents a partnership among governments, the private sector, and worldwide communities. The fund awarded its first round of grants to 36 countries later in that same year.[5] The establishment of this fund, and the inclusion of the control of HIV/AIDS and other diseases as one of eight measurable UN Millennium Development Goals in 2000 (United Nations, 2000), underscore the perceived importance of infectious diseases to global development prospects.
- In 2003, leaders from the 21 members of the Asia-Pacific Economic Cooperation (APEC) forum, including the U.S. President, endorsed a new health security initiative that included a provision for infectious disease surveillance and response (see APEC, 2003).

Despite the renewed attention to global infectious disease since the 1990s, efforts to significantly improve global surveillance have been only partly successful: In the late 1990s, the IOM asserted, "The necessary information and communications technology are available, yet no formal infectious-disease surveillance system exists on a global scale" (Howson, Fineberg, and Bloom, 1998, p. 588). In a follow-up report in 2003, the IOM noted the ongoing nature of the problem: "Health ministries may generate health reports, but the data are generally unreliable. Such numbers have been used as the basis for broad policy recommendations; if the numbers are incorrect, however, the resulting policies can be damaging" (Smolinski, Hamburg, and Lederberg, 2003, p. 154).

Global Infectious Disease Surveillance

Global disease surveillance is conducted through a loose framework of formal, informal, and ad hoc arrangements that the U.S. General Accounting Office, now the U.S. Government Accountability Office (GAO), has characterized as a "network of networks" (U.S. General

---

[5] For information about the Global Fund to Fight AIDS, Tuberculosis and Malaria, visit its Web site, http://www.theglobalfund.org/ (online as of June 12, 2006).

Accounting Office, 2000a). Historically, surveillance systems have been developed mainly to address specific diseases. Those that are targeted for eradication or elimination, such as polio, tend to receive sustained financial and technical support, while surveillance for other diseases, including emerging diseases, has received limited support (U.S. General Accounting Office, 2001). The lack of adequate sustained support for surveillance adds to the challenge of controlling emerging diseases.

Surveillance systems in all countries suffer from a number of common constraints, but these constraints are more prevalent in the poorest countries, where annual per capita expenditure on all aspects of health care is less than 30 U.S. dollars, representing 2–3 percent of these nations' gross domestic product (United Nations Development Programme, 2005). The most common constraints are shortages of human and material resources: Trained personnel and laboratory equipment are lacking in many cases (U.S. General Accounting Office, 2001). Poor coordination of surveillance activities also constrains global disease surveillance. This poor coordination is caused by multiple reporting systems, unclear lines of authority, and incomplete participation by affected countries (U.S. General Accounting Office, 2001), resulting in knowledge gaps about putative outbreaks. Therefore, shortcomings in surveillance reporting of infectious disease seem to exist for two main reasons: Some nations are either unable or unwilling to report.

Recent Improvements in Global Disease Surveillance

In 2000, the WHO formalized the Global Outbreak Alert and Response Network (GOARN), which links over 100 laboratory and reporting networks. Development of GOARN began in 1997. GOARN relies on a Canadian-developed system known as the Global Public Health Intelligence Network (GPHIN), which includes software that actively gathers disease information from Web sites, news wires, newspapers, public health email services, and electronic discussion groups; processes the information centrally in Canada; and then sends alerts to the WHO for verification. GPHIN has identified more than 40 percent of the outbreaks subsequently verified by the WHO (Heymann, 2003). GPHIN is beneficial because it can identify possible outbreaks more quickly than can traditional systems, in which case reports must be passed up from the local level to subnational and national governments, and ultimately reported to the WHO. However, GPHIN can only identify rumors of outbreaks where they might be reported in the media or on discussion Web sites, and some diseases occur in areas so remote that they are not detected by the sources that GPHIN searches, or in countries using foreign languages not currently compatible with GPHIN.

Updated International Health Regulations

The World Health Organization has recently revised its International Health Regulations (IHR), which govern the responsibilities of member states and the WHO in response to selected infectious disease threats of international concern. This was the result of a long process and an even longer history of global governance related to infectious diseases. In this section, we highlight the history and recent developments with respect to these IHR.

In 1896, the International Sanitary Conference agreed that there was a need for international health surveillance (Zacher, 1999). That year marked the beginning of cooperative surveillance for global infectious disease. The Organisation Internationale d'Hygiène Publique was established in Paris in 1907 to gather and share information on disease outbreaks among participating countries (Cash and Narasimhan, 2000). Eventually requiring the reporting of plague, cholera, yellow fever, smallpox, relapsing fever, and typhus, the impetus for this agreement was that Europe feared that these diseases would enter from poorer countries where they were most prevalent (Fidler, 1997).

The Organisation Internationale d'Hygiène Publique was replaced by the WHO, which was created in 1948 and issued its International Sanitary Regulations in 1951. These regulations were renamed the International Health Regulations in 1969 and were later revised in 1981. The 1981 regulations required member nations to notify the WHO within 24 hours of an outbreak of plague, cholera, or yellow fever. However, the IHR applied only to nations that were members of the WHO and only to those three diseases. The WHO, lacking strong enforcement powers, has relied mostly on international persuasion to ensure compliance. Nations have not always complied (Heymann and Rodier, 1998), fearing the economic consequences of preventive actions and reduced travel and trade, even though the reporting of outbreaks often triggers international assistance.

Although the revision process began before the 2003 SARS outbreak in China, the SARS experience was undoubtedly on the minds of the 192 member nations of the World Health Assembly when they ratified the revised IHR in May 2005 (see World Health Organization, 2005).[6] The revision process began when the World Health Assembly, dissatisfied with the limitations of the current IHR, endorsed a resolution in 1995 to revise them. These efforts failed, but the Assembly renewed its resolve to revise the IHR through a new resolution in 2003,[7] culminating in a substantially revised agreement, a legally binding treaty that it endorsed in 2005 (see World Health Organization, 2005). The revised regulations include an expanded list of diseases that member nations are required to report to the WHO. The IHR also include a decision matrix for nations to determine whether an outbreak—due to a disease on the expanded list or a newly emerged disease—is significant enough to require reporting (i.e., a "public health emergency of international concern") with new attention paid to the propensity of disease to be spread via modern travel methods. Importantly, given the SARS and avian influenza experiences, the IHR require nations to respond to requests for verification from the WHO, whether the WHO learns of a putative outbreak from the affected nation or via other means, such as GPHIN (World Health Organization, 2005). Cash and Narasimhan (2000), writing while the IHR revisions were being discussed, suggested that the expansion of the number of reportable diseases in the revised IHR could increase the use of trade and travel restrictions in an attempt to prevent the spread of infectious agents across borders. In that paper, they provide examples of how "overreaction" to reported outbreaks has had significant consequences for affected nations (e.g., see the discussion about plague in India in Chapter Three), and they suggest that the IHR can be used to prevent such overreactions, in part by preventing the rapid spread of inaccurate reports.

---

[6] This revision is also timely, given the increasing threat of a human influenza pandemic arising from avian influenza that is currently circulating in Asia and elsewhere.

[7] For the text of the resolution to revise the IHR, Resolution 56.28, see World Health Assembly (2003).

Because the revised IHR emphasize timely disclosure of outbreaks by affected countries, an important component is the assurance that technical assistance will be provided by the WHO and its member states to help both strengthen surveillance and respond to outbreaks of emerging disease threats of international concern. The revised regulations are aimed to improve global disease detection and control through public health capacity and compliance.

Summary

Globalization and the modern-day threats of infectious diseases have kept these diseases on the public policy agenda into the 21st century. Recent policy and programming responses by both the United States and the broader global community provide the context from which we examine the three research questions addressed in this study.

CHAPTER THREE

Addressing a New Paradigm: Infectious Disease and National Security

Our first research question asks how the emerging link between global infectious disease and U.S. national security has been perceived and acted upon across government sectors. This chapter begins with a section describing the evolution of this new paradigm, the effects of infectious disease on security, the implications of a biosecurity policy orientation to natural disease outbreaks, and the implications for global disease reporting. This chapter then summarizes a number of recent U.S. security initiatives addressing infectious diseases. The final section presents the views of stakeholders we interviewed regarding their perceptions of the link between infectious disease and national security.

Infectious Disease and Security

Evolving Security Concepts

Traditional views of the association between infectious disease and security have often focused on the effect of health on military success (for example, see Szreter, 2003). In fact, many health discoveries that were made in the course of efforts to protect armies ultimately benefited other populations as well. For example, discoveries made near the turn of the 20th century, including the tracing of the natural history of diseases such as yellow fever and malaria, were studied initially in an effort to protect military forces (Berlinguer, 2003), and World War II provided the impetus to mass-produce penicillin.

Similarly, the U.S. State Department has speculated that disease will emerge as a "conflict starter," and possibly even a "war outcome determinant" (see, for example, Center for Strategic International Studies, 2000, and U.S. Department of State, 1995). The relationship between disease and warfare is as old as war itself. Indeed, disease among armies has long been a contributing factor to military outcomes, and warfare has contributed to the spread of disease.[1] Following World War II, and based upon the institutions established at the end of that war, worldwide perceptions of national security were largely restricted to the military defense of territorial borders and interests; these perceptions were not much different from concepts of security prior to that war (Rothschild, 1995). The association of disease with warfare parallels traditional views of national security, i.e., armed protection of a nation's borders and inter-

---

[1] A complete discussion of this subject is beyond the scope of this study; more information can be found in Gabriel and Metz (1992) and Smallman-Raynor and Cliff (2004).

ests. Similarly, traditional views of the relationship between disease and security have focused on the threat of disease spreading across borders. However, increasing worldwide attention has recently been paid to a broader issue: the effect of infectious disease on other concepts of security.

These newer concepts include the recognition of the inherent benefit of health: "[H]ealth itself is a power, a fundamental capacity for the development or maintenance of all other capacities" (Berlinguer, 2003, p. 57). This view has been extended from the individual to the state: when nations recognize that investment in health can improve the health of a nation's population, advance its economy, and "promote humane values and moral leadership in a world of opportunities and profound health needs" (Howson, Fineberg, and Bloom, 1998, p. 590). This view illustrates the newly evolving concept of "human security." In 1994, the UN Development Programme wrote of a transition "from nuclear security to human security," meaning safety from "hunger, disease and repression" (United Nations Development Programme, 1994, p. 23). Shortly thereafter, the UN Secretary-General gave formal voice to a development that had been more than a decade in the making, calling for a "conceptual breakthrough," going "beyond armed territorial security" and protecting the "security of people in their homes, jobs, and communities" (Rothschild, 1995, quoting then–UN Secretary-General Boutros Boutros-Ghali).

The UN established an independent international commission on human security in 2001, mandated to clarify the concept of human security for global policy and action (Chen and Narasimhan, 2003). Chen and Narasimhan (2003) assert that "a new people-centered paradigm, with its policy and operational implications, can complement and strengthen state security to protect people in an unstable and interconnected world," and "control of global infections is not possible without surveillance, control and response linked to international trade, migration, and movements" (p. 11). The UN commission produced a working definition of human security: "The objective of human security is to safeguard the vital core of human lives from critical pervasive threats while promoting long-term human flourishing" (Chen and Narasimhan, 2003, p. 4). In its final report, the commission asserted that "[g]lobal health is both essential and instrumental to achieving human security," and "illness, disability and avoidable death are 'critical pervasive threats' to human security" (Commission on Human Security, 2003, p. 96).

Effects of Infectious Disease on Security

The discussion of human security versus older, traditional ideas of security is useful in understanding the moral values with which the global community appears to approach the importance of health today. However, it remains somewhat intangible, leaving firm associations between health (including infectious disease) and security incompletely defined. As Chen and Narasimhan (2003) point out, "health and human security are fundamentally valued in all societies, but their connections and interdependencies are not well understood." Nonetheless, some authors assert a solid association between health and security, at least for the United States: "National security and public health experts agree that infectious diseases pose a substantial direct and indirect threat to U.S. interests" (U.S. Government Accounting Office, 2000a, p. 2). Such assertions are based on a growing body of evidence that associates infectious disease with effects that may ultimately threaten both human and national concepts of security. As Brower and Chalk (2003) conclude, there is a definite link between infectious disease and security: Disease can affect individuals and also weaken public confidence in a government's ability to respond; they have an adverse economic impact, undermine a state's social order, catalyze regional instability, and pose a strategic threat through bioterrorism or biowarfare.

Compelling arguments have been made linking infectious disease to conditions that logically can affect security. These conditions include those mentioned by Brower and Chalk (2003), and others that have been argued by numerous other authors. The following is a summary of research that has associated specific effects of infectious disease with threats to security.

Direct Mortality and Morbidity. The most obvious effect of disease that may result in the instability of a nation or region is the toll of some diseases that have high mortality rates. Such diseases, especially if highly prevalent, can pose a direct risk to a nation's security by threatening to sicken and kill a significant portion of a country's population (Heymann, 2003; Price-Smith, 2002), and a disease that targets sectors of a population that are relied upon for production and military protection can be particularly ominous (see also Chyba, 1998; Enemark, 2004; Frist, 2005; and White House, 2004). HIV/AIDS is a disease often cited in this regard.

Economic Loss. As detailed in examples later in this chapter, an outbreak of disease—or even the perceived threat of an outbreak—can have significant repercussions on trade and travel for the affected nation. The economic effects of infectious diseases—whether endemic, e.g., malaria, or epidemic, e.g., cholera—can be devastating. As just one example, it has been estimated that Africa's gross domestic product would be nearly one-third higher if malaria alone had been eliminated several decades ago (U.S. General Accounting Office, 2001). Many of these effects are indirect (e.g., loss of productivity and commerce), but there are also direct economic costs (e.g., culling of animal herds and medical costs of treating humans) that may affect security and relationships between nations in need and those able to provide assistance to control outbreaks. (For examples of both direct and indirect costs, see Brower and Chalk, 2003; Cash and Narasimhan, 2000; Enemark, 2004; Frist, 2005; Heymann, 2003; United Nations Security Council, 2000; U.S. General Accounting Office, 2001; U.S. National Intelligence Council, 2000; White House, 2004; and Wilson, 2003a.) In addition, the UN estimated in 2002 that $20 billion would be needed by 2007 to provide adequate prevention and care for populations affected by HIV/AIDS in low- and middle-income countries (UNAIDS, 2002; see also World Health Organization, 2002).

Social and Governmental Disruption. It has been documented that infectious diseases cause significant social disruption through fear and anxiety about a disease (based on accurate or inaccurate information), the loss of people in key social positions due to illness or death, discrimination against groups affected by a disease, and the loss of the majority of (or entire) specific demographic groups. (For examples of social disruption, see Chyba, 1998; Elbe, 2002; Enemark, 2004; Heymann, 2003; Ostergard, 2002; Shisana, Zungu-Dirwayi, and Shisana, 2003; Store, Welch, and Chen, 2003; UNAIDS, 2004; U.S. National Intelligence Council, 2000; White House, 2004; and Wilson, 2003a.) Consider HIV/AIDS: In 2003, there were 3 million new infections in sub-Saharan Africa (UNAIDS, 2002, 2004). Since it was first diagnosed in 1981, HIV/AIDS has accounted for approximately 20 million deaths worldwide. Between 34.6 and 42.3 million people were living with HIV/AIDS in 2003, and the disease had orphaned approximately 12 million children in sub-Saharan Africa alone (UNAIDS, 2004). Half of new infections occur among 15- to 24-year-olds (UNAIDS, 2004), a traditionally productive segment of society. The reduction of this demographic group can lead to economic loss due to reduced productivity, but it also represents the loss of a core group of parents, social leaders, and key members of society, such as teachers and soldiers. Ministries of defense in some sub-Saharan African countries report HIV prevalence averages of 20–40 percent in their armed services, potentially affecting their military capabilities (UNAIDS, 2002).

Not surprisingly, HIV/AIDS in sub-Saharan Africa has been associated with the destabilization of infrastructures needed for governance (Heymann, 2003), as well as with the disruption of cohesion and stability of families, communities, and nation-states (Heymann, 2003; Shisana, Zungu-Dirwayi, and Shisana, 2003; Store, Welch, and Chen, 2003). As a society is degraded by infectious disease, its populace may lose confidence in a government that seems unable to control the disease. Such a loss in confidence, it has been asserted, results in a degradation of a government's legitimacy and may lead to increased migration or increased vulnerability to economic or military competition from other nations. (For examples of government disruption and instability, see Brower and Chalk, 2003; Enemark, 2004; Heymann, 2003; Huang, 2003; Ostergard, 2002; United Nations Security Council, 2000; U.S. National Intelligence Council, 2000; and Wilson, 2003a.)

Implications of a Biodefense Orientation for Natural Disease Outbreaks
Heymann (2003) points out that the response of industrialized countries has not been commensurate with the views of various organizations, such as the UN and the U.S. National Intelligence Council, that infectious diseases pose a threat to international security. During the 1990s, it remained unclear whether or not infectious diseases were seriously considered in the national security strategies of developed countries. That changed after the attacks on the United States in September and October 2001, and the newly perceived risk of bioterrorism, "immediately raised the infectious disease threat to the level of a high priority security imperative worthy of attention in defense and intelligence circles" (Heymann, 2003, p. 105).

While there is growing recognition in recent U.S. policy that improved preparation for bioattacks (i.e., bioterrorism) on the U.S. homeland can also result in improved surveillance for and response to naturally occurring disease outbreaks and vice versa, it is obvious that many of the initiatives since 2001 (described later in this chapter) have been focused on the former. There has been some debate about whether preparation for both events is complementary or whether a focus on bioattacks distracts from surveillance of naturally occurring disease, or vice versa. Brower and Chalk (2003) suggested that the United States expends considerable policy attention and resources to defend against "relatively unlikely" scenarios, such as a large-scale bioterrorist attack, concluding that "[r]esponses to more commonly occurring and currently more taxing natural outbreaks remain relatively overlooked and underfunded" (p. xix).

In recent years, the public health and homeland security communities seem to have come to a realization that the public health infrastructure for infectious diseases in fact also underpins the public health aspects of bioterrorism detection and early response. It seems to many that the only rational way to defend the world against a bioterrorist attack is to have a central principle of global public health security and to strengthen the capacity to detect and contain naturally occurring outbreaks (Heymann, 2003). Some authors have argued compellingly that public health surveillance for emerging diseases and preparedness for and detection of biological terrorism are strongly related (see, for example, Chyba, 1998). Presentations by the United States and other countries at the July 19–24, 2004, Meeting of Experts, held during the Biological and Toxins Weapon Convention, addressed surveillance and mitigation within this very framework, i.e., bioterrorism detection and early response relying in large part on the underlying public health infrastructure.[2]

The themes of the 2002 U.S. National Security Strategy include defeating terrorism and tyranny, as well as fostering the spread of freedom worldwide. U.S. experts recognized that infectious diseases pose a substantial obstacle to U.S. efforts to encourage economic growth and betterment in the lives of the poor in the developing world (U.S. General Accounting Office, 2000a). For example, the National Security Strategy recognizes that the United States' strategic priority of combating global terror is threatened by disease (as well as war and desperate poverty) in Africa. While a significant focus of the strategy is defense against terrorist attacks in the United States, it also acknowledges that investments to defend against such attacks also present related opportunities: "Our medical system will be strengthened to manage not just bioterror, but all infectious diseases and mass-casualty dangers" (White House, 2002, pp. 6–7).

Infectious Disease, Security, and Disease Reporting

Given the potential consequences of infectious disease on a country's international trade and economy (and, by extension, security), it is not surprising that some countries choose not to report disease outbreaks, or at least to delay their reporting. Such decisions can have global effects.

With the major exception of HIV/AIDS, newly identified infectious diseases have not had a large effect on global infectious disease mortality, but new diseases are of concern due to their large numbers of casualties and high profile (Wilson, 2003a). While this observation is not necessarily predictive of the mortality caused by future emerging and reemerging diseases, the visibility of some diseases has caused anxiety that is sometimes out of proportion with the actual risk. Examples include plague in India (Wilson, 1995a) and Ebola in sub-Saharan Africa, which has emerged periodically since 1976, even though no scientific evidence suggests a serious risk of global spread of Ebola (other than through bioterrorism) (Wilson, 2003a). It should be noted that the level of anxiety caused by some diseases is, in fact, commensurate with the scale of their actual medical and societal effects. HIV/AIDS is one such example. In other cases, an increased level of anxiety can make permissible intensive and large-scale public health measures that may not have been possible previously, as was seen in the global response to SARS and the public acceptance of containment measures.

---

[2] Melinda Moore, an author of this report, was a U.S. delegate to this meeting. The meeting report is available at http://www.opbw.org/new_process/mx2004/bwc_msp.2004_mx_3_E.pdf, and a related press release is available at http://www2.unog.ch/news2/documents/newsen/dc04029e.htm (both as of October 31, 2005).

Nonetheless, anxiety associated with such diseases, as well as subsequent legitimate public health intervention measures, has sometimes resulted in significant economic effects, including lost trade and tourism and the required culling of animal herds. Such economic effects or other unfavorable treatment by the world community have been a disincentive for countries to report outbreaks (see Cash and Narasimhan, 2000, and Fidler, 1997), yet they can have an important net benefit on public health and the global economy.[3] As such, a disinclination of countries to report and respond appropriately to disease outbreaks poses a dangerous prospect in the face of a potential worldwide disease outbreak, such as pandemic influenza.

International knowledge about infectious disease outbreaks, whether reported by the affected country or otherwise discovered, can have significant negative economic consequences through decreased trade and travel. Cash and Narasimhan (2000), in a study on the impediments of global infectious disease surveillance, found that "current guidelines and regulations on emerging and re-emerging infectious diseases do not sufficiently take into account the fact that when developing countries report outbreaks they often derive few benefits and suffer disproportionately heavy social and economic consequences" (p. 1358). Their article presented two cases to support this conclusion: plague in India and cholera in South America. The illustrative case of plague in India is summarized below.

Plague in India. In September 1994, a hospital in Surat, India, admitted seven patients with pneumonia-like symptoms. Rather than waiting a week for laboratory confirmation of plague-like bacilli from patient samples, Indian officials declared an outbreak of plague. This decision may have also reflected a conservative public health approach, prompted by the fact that India's public health laboratory infrastructure had eroded in the previous decade. Unfortunately, like many other places in the world, India lacked a robust diagnostic capability to confirm or rule out plague infections rapidly and confidently.[4] Within three days, as many as 500,000 people fled Surat and the surrounding area, reacting to media reports of a plague outbreak. A low-threshold case definition of plague was adopted, and any persons showing respiratory symptoms were quarantined. Schools were closed, cargo was fumigated against rodents, flea controls were implemented, and antibiotics were administered to individuals who were presumed to be exposed. A WHO investigative team concluded that these measures were excessive. After implementing control measures, India declared the epidemic controlled in early October 1994, and the WHO concurred at the end of October of that year. In the end, either no (Cash and Narasimhan, 2000) or few cases of plague were confirmed on the basis of WHO bacterial standards.[5]

Even without a scientific confirmation of a plague outbreak, press reports were estimating the magnitude of the outbreak, and some nations responded by stopping air travel to and from India. Although the WHO requested that no travel or trade restrictions be imposed, Bangladesh, Oman, Qatar, and the United Arab Emirates stopped importing all Indian food;

---

[3] Economic benefits of local intervention measures may be realized outside the affected country by preventing the international spread of disease, thus avoiding increased costs of additional, widespread animal culling and reduced trade and travel among other countries, for example.

[4] Ruth Berkelman, Emory University, personal communication, March 14, 2006.

[5] Ruth Berkelman, Emory University, personal communication, March 14, 2006.

Bangladesh halted all goods and people from crossing its border with India. Canada, France, Germany, Italy, the United Kingdom, and the United States issued travel warnings. Italy placed an embargo on all Indian goods, and Sweden canceled all textile shipments (Cash and Narasimhan, 2000, citing media reports).

The world reaction to the suspected—but unconfirmed—plague outbreak had a significant impact on India's economy. In 1994, India's trade deficit doubled in comparison to the year before (Fidler et al., 1997). Overall, losses associated with the reported outbreak have been estimated at $2 billion (Levy and Gage, 1999), though long-term loss projections may be higher (Cash and Narasimhan, 2000). Cash and Narasimhan (2000) comment that other countries, observing the price that India paid, will probably be more reluctant to report similar outbreaks in the future. These authors observe that "[p]aradoxically, when a country reports an outbreak, the international community may benefit relatively little, whereas the reporting country itself may suffer great losses" (Cash and Narasimhan, 2000, p. 1364). They conclude that, if the interests of reporting countries are not protected, they are "likely to continue trying to conceal epidemics, and the goals of global surveillance are unlikely to be fully achieved" (p. 1365).

In addition to economic consequences, countries may also be unwilling to report outbreaks or may overstate their preparedness for reasons of international prestige. For example, nearly every country initially denied or minimized the prevalence of HIV/AIDS within its borders (U.S. National Intelligence Council, 2000), partly because of the social and sexual stigma surrounding the disease. There is some evidence that a desire to protect its international image was a factor in China's reluctance to report an outbreak of SARS in 2003, although the economic consequences of that outbreak were also significant, as discussed below.

SARS in China and Beyond. The world experience of the 2003 SARS outbreak that began in China underscored the consequences of a nation failing to report an outbreak in a timely and accurate manner. The earliest human case of SARS is thought to have occurred in the Guangdong province, China, in November 2002. It apparently spread to humans through the slaughter of infected animals in unsanitary and crowded markets (Osterholm, 2005). The outbreak came to the attention of Chinese health officials as early as a month later (Huang, 2003). Because Chinese law regarding the handling of public health–related information mandated that information about such outbreaks be classified as a state secret before being announced by the Ministry of Health, any physician or journalist who reported on the disease would risk accusation of leaking state secrets. Therefore, although the Chinese Ministry of Health was informed of the outbreak in January 2003, a news blackout persisted until February of that year (Huang, 2003), and the provincial government did not show evidence of taking the public health threat seriously and responding in a timely and appropriate manner. A contagious disease coupled with government inaction took a significant toll on the frontline responders—health care providers (Huang, 2003). By the end of February 2003, nearly half the 900 cases in the Guangdong province city of Guangzhou were among health care workers (Pomfret, 2003). With a blackout on reporting about the disease within China, let alone the rest of the world, carriers of the disease traveled to other cities, provinces, and countries, perhaps oblivious to the risk that they could spread the disease. The SARS outbreak was eventually noticed by the WHO. Finally, WHO experts were invited to China, where they were given access to

Guangdong only after waiting eight days in Beijing. They were not allowed to inspect military hospitals in Beijing for another week, and by that time the disease had already spread internationally (Huang, 2003).

In addition to the delay in reporting to the WHO, the information provided by Chinese officials was suspect, perhaps because they tried to avoid damage to China's international image, as well as economic consequences that may have resulted from international reactions. When the WHO issued the first travel advisory in its 55-year history, recommending that people not visit Hong Kong or Guangdong, the Chinese health minister promised that China was safe and that the outbreak was under control. Earlier, the minister announced that only 12 cases of SARS had been identified in Beijing when in fact in the city's No. 309 People's Liberation Army Hospital alone there were 60 SARS patients (Huang, 2003).

By the end of 2003, SARS had killed 774 people and infected over 8,000 people in 29 countries (World Health Organization, 2003). The initial lack of cooperation from officials in China may have contributed to this spread, but the extent to which it did so is unclear and may never be known (U.S. Government Accountability Office, 2004). It is also unclear the extent to which this initial lack of cooperation affected the overall economic consequence of the outbreak, estimated at $11 billion to $18 billion (U.S. Government Accountability Office, 2004). What is clearer is that SARS highlighted the importance of prompt and accurate reporting of disease outbreaks.

As summarized above and illustrated by the examples of plague in India and SARS in China and beyond, numerous authors have suggested that infectious disease can have significant effects on security, for individuals, nations, and the world. Because some of these effects are manifest in international relationships (e.g., travel and commerce), nations are caught in a difficult position when they experience an infectious disease outbreak. Reporting an outbreak can initiate a response internally and from outside the nation, which may result in timely and effective disease-control actions that mitigate social disruption, government destabilization, and loss of productivity within the affected country. On the other hand, a nation reporting a disease outbreak may experience disruption of trade and travel and suffer economic losses related to intervention measures (e.g., culling of bird flocks in the case of avian influenza). The resulting economic effects may be disproportionately large in the affected nation, in comparison with the effects on its multiple trading partners. Faced with this possibility, an affected country may be reluctant to report an outbreak, given the current lack of protection against (what may be unnecessary) international reactions. Policymakers hope that improved global disease surveillance and the recently revised International Health Regulations, both described in Chapter Two, may help mitigate this problem.

Infectious Disease and Recent U.S. National Security Initiatives

While global infectious disease began to receive increased policy attention in the United States beginning in the 1990s, the attacks of September 11, 2001, and the anthrax attacks of the following month, focused new attention on preparedness for detecting and responding to bioterrorism attacks. The U.S. Department of Homeland Security (DHS), which was formed in response to the 2001 attacks, is the integrator of numerous new initiatives. The remainder of this chapter summarizes efforts to operationalize the new paradigm linking infectious diseases to national security, specifically the policy decisions following the attacks of 2001 and the resulting organizations and initiatives. These organizations and initiatives either build upon or supplement already-established systems for infectious disease surveillance.

On June 12, 2002, Congress passed the Public Health Security and Bioterrorism Preparedness and Response Act (Public Law 107-188), requiring specific actions related to bioterrorism preparedness and response (U.S. Government Accountability Office, 2005). The law required the establishment of an integrated communications and surveillance network among federal, state, and local public health officials, as well as public and private health-related laboratories and hospitals. The act pertained to bioterrorism on the U.S. homeland, but the intended improvements are also useful for detecting and responding to natural infectious disease outbreaks.

Concerned primarily about the potential risk to the United States from the deliberate use of biological agents, the President instructed federal departments and agencies to review their efforts and find ways to improve security against bioattacks in the United States. The result of this review was a joint strategy, embodied in Homeland Security Presidential Directive (HSPD) 10 and National Security Presidential Directive (NSPD) 33, *Biodefense for the 21st Century*, collectively (White House, 2004). HPSD-10/NSPD-33 gives DHS the authority to coordinate a sustained effort against biological weapons threats, and it is based on four essential pillars (White House, 2004; Vitko, 2005):

1. *Threat awareness,* including biological weapons–related intelligence, risk assessments, and anticipation of future threats
2. *Prevention and protection,* including proactive prevention and infrastructure protection
3. *Surveillance and detection,* including attack warning and attribution
4. *Response and recovery.*

HSPD-10/NSPD-33 addresses the threat of deliberate use of a biological agent. While recognizing that "disease outbreaks, whether natural or deliberate, respect no geographic or political borders" (White House 2004), in only one instance does the document note that preparation for an intentional outbreak can also benefit the broader risk of natural infectious disease: "Private, local, and state capabilities are being augmented by and coordinated with Federal assets, to provide layered defenses against biological weapons attacks. These improvements will complement and enhance our defense against emerging or reemerging natural infectious diseases" (White House, 2004).

HSPD-10/NSPD-33 spurred the development of a number of specific, related initiatives. For example, the Office of Science and Technology Policy considers the Biosurveillance Initiative to be composed of three key initiatives: BioWatch, BioSense, and the National Biosurveillance Integration System (NBIS) (Office of Science and Technology Policy, 2005). Also stemming from HSPD-10/NSPD-33 are two initiatives related to research on and procurement of medical countermeasures directed mostly against terrorism threats: BioShield and the National Biodefense Analysis and Countermeasures Center (NBACC). The following sections summarize initiatives created by the U.S. government since 2001.

BioWatch

BioWatch is an early warning environmental monitoring system that collects air samples from multiple locations in approximately 30 U.S. cities deemed to be at high risk of an intentional attack with biological agents (Office of Science and Technology Policy, 2005). BioWatch laboratories, all of which are part of the CDC's Laboratory Response Network (LRN), test the samples for selected agents and use a reporting system to send data to the CDC in order to support response to a potential outbreak (U.S. Government Accountability Office, 2005). BioWatch is a cooperative effort of DHS, the CDC's LRN, and the Environmental Protection Agency (Office of Science and Technology Policy, 2005).

BioSense

Project BioSense was initiated by the CDC in fiscal year 2003 to improve the United States' ability to monitor human health events.[6] This nationwide system monitors the health status of American populations by analyzing diagnoses from ambulatory care sites, laboratory testing orders, and over-the-counter drug sales, in addition to other data sources. Monitored human disease trends can be integrated with environmental sampling data from Project BioWatch to present coordinated information to support response efforts (Office of Science and Technology Policy, 2005). However, the GAO has reported that BioSense is not widely used by state and local public health officials, primarily because of limitations in the data it collects (U.S. Government Accountability Office, 2005).

National Biosurveillance Integration System

A nascent government-wide system managed and coordinated by DHS, NBIS is intended to combine multiple data streams from sector-specific agencies—those with health, environmental, agricultural, and intelligence data—to provide all stakeholders with broad situational awareness that is expected to allow for earlier detection of events and to facilitate coordinated response (U.S. Government Accountability Office, 2005). The main goal of NBIS is to collect, assemble, and analyze a wide range of relevant information and make such information available to government stakeholders in a timely and reliable fashion. Once fully operational, NBIS will collect data from DHS sources and other U.S. government agencies within a common platform and combine those data with environmental and intelligence data. Analysts from DHS will work together with analysts on DHS and NBIS detail from other federal agencies to process this information and present "situational awareness" to the DHS Homeland

---

[6] Since the completion of data collection for this study, BioSense was revised and is now referred to as BioSense Real-Time (BioSense RT). This system is intended to receive a broad set of data directly from health care organizations in real time, with a special emphasis on information from emergency rooms, where people are most likely to go during an outbreak. It is also intended to provide simultaneous access to these data by all jurisdictional levels of public health (hospital, city, county, state, national). The emphasis of Biosense RT is less on the early detection of an event and more on how the health care system is able to respond by allocating available resources (see Caldwell, 2006).

Security Operations Center (Morr, 2005) and an Interagency Incident Management Group, as described in the National Response Plan (U.S. Department of Homeland Security, 2004).

NBIS is intended to help meet the HSPD-10/NSPD-33 call for "creating a national bio-awareness system that will permit the recognition of a biological attack at the earliest possible moment" (White House, 2004). Like other new DHS initiatives, NBIS was originally intended to focus only on intentional disease outbreaks (i.e., bioattacks) (Vitko, 2005). In fact, all of the DHS initiatives are intended to fit within the department's "niche" by focusing exclusively on a homeland-directed attack (Morr, 2005), but officials at NBIS acknowledged that, because it is often difficult to determine initially whether or not an outbreak is deliberately caused, NBIS will also be useful in providing early warning of naturally occurring outbreaks. Further, unlike most other DHS initiatives, NBIS is more international in scope, though its intent is ultimately domestic protection. (NBACC also considers international information, including intelligence, to identify material threats.)

A key component of NBIS is software that actively probes the Internet for reports or rumors of disease events; the software systematically searches over 1 million sites each day. There is some evidence that this software has identified recent outbreaks significantly earlier than other systems have.

The DHS Science and Technology Directorate developed the NBIS system requirements and then transferred the initiative to the Directorate for Information Analysis and Infrastructure Protection in December 2004 for implementation. The genesis of NBIS appears to be a comprehensive 2003 study of the ability of the United States to rapidly detect bioattacks. A series of interagency meetings culminated in a report in December 2004 that marked the end of the requirements-determination process and the start of the implementation process. (The December 2004 report was not made available to RAND.) As of this writing, NBIS is under development, and its staff of analysts and information systems are being established in phases. NBIS officials intend for NBIS to serve as the "eyes and ears" of the nation for indicators and warnings that prompt early detection of a disease outbreak, whether natural or deliberate in origin; it is not designed to replace existing agencies' responsibilities for response, risk assessment, or forensic attribution.

BioShield

Signed into law by President Bush in July 2004, Project BioShield is an initiative to speed the development and procurement of new medical countermeasures against chemical, biological, radiological, and nuclear terrorist threats. The President committed $5.6 billion over ten years to accelerate development and stockpile vaccines, drugs, and diagnostic aids to fight anthrax, smallpox, and other potential threat agents (Office of Science and Technology Policy, 2005). The procurement of these products is supported by work at the NBACC.

National Biodefense Analysis and Countermeasures Center

In accordance with HSPD-10/NSPD-33, DHS requested and received appropriated funding, beginning in fiscal year 2003, for the construction of NBACC, a biodefense facility dedicated to homeland security activities. As of this writing, NBACC research programs are operating while the facility itself is being constructed within the National Interagency Biodefense Campus at Fort Detrick, Maryland. Other agencies on this campus will include the Department of Health and Human Services' National Institutes of Health (specifically, its National Institute of Allergy and Infectious Diseases) and Centers for Disease Control and Prevention, the Department of Agriculture's Agricultural Research Service and Foreign Disease–Weed Science Research Institute, and the Department of Defense's (DoD's) U.S. Army Medical Research Institute of Infectious Diseases (U.S. Department of Homeland Security, 2005). Coordination of NBACC is performed by various interagency committees at different levels of seniority.

NBACC principally comprises two component parts: the National Bioforensic Analysis Center and the Biological Threat Characterization Center (McQueary, 2005). A third component, the Biodefense Knowledge Center (BKC), was dedicated in September 2004 and is located at the Department of Energy's Los Alamos National Laboratory (Shea, 2005). Programs undertaken by NBACC are currently conducted through partnerships and agreements with federal and private institutions (Martinez-Lopez, 2004); for example, the BKC draws upon the Lawrence Livermore National Laboratory and three DHS Centers of Excellence, at the University of Minnesota, the University of Southern California, and Texas A&M University (U.S. Department of Energy, 2004). The mission of the NBACC is to understand current and future biological threats, assess vulnerabilities and determine potential consequences, and provide a national capability for conducting forensic analysis of evidence from biocrimes and terrorism (Albright, 2005). This mission will support the procurement of countermeasures under Project BioShield by assessing potential bioterrorism agents as "material threats." Project BioShield requires that the Secretary of Homeland Security determine whether such a "material threat" exists before countermeasures can be taken (Gottron, 2003). NBACC provides a formal threat assessment every two years; the first is due in 2006 (Vitko, 2005). The scope of this first assessment has been agreed upon by the interagency Biodefense Policy Coordinating Committee, which is cochaired by the Homeland Security Council and the National Security Council. It will address 29 biological agents, evaluate the vulnerability of the United States to threats posed by these agents, and consider the potential consequences of any such attacks (Vitko, 2005).

Department of Defense Initiatives

DoD's Walter Reed Army Institute of Research oversees the identification of possible biological threats to populations worldwide through the joint Global Emerging Infections System (GEIS), which draws upon overseas military medical research facilities to help monitor disease, and the Electronic Surveillance System for the Early Notification of Community-Based Epidemics (ESSENCE), which uses data-mining techniques to identify unusually high rates of specified clinical syndromes. Additionally, DoD is deploying an improved Joint Biological Agent Identification and Diagnosis System to rapidly identify biological threat agents (Office of Science and Technology Policy, 2005).

Summary

A new paradigm has evolved that links infectious disease to security, recognizing the broad effects of disease on societies. One implication of this paradigm is that nations may take actions against one another to prevent infectious disease from reaching their borders. In some cases, these actions may be of some global benefit (i.e., in preventing disease spread), but their effects may result in disproportionate costs to a nation experiencing an outbreak. This situation can present disincentives to disease reporting by nations, even if the nation possesses the capability to do so. In recognition of this emerging paradigm, the United States has recently undertaken a number of initiatives to address infectious disease, including a DHS initiative, NBIS, intended to detect outbreaks worldwide and to provide information to all relevant federal stakeholders.

Many stakeholders we interviewed acknowledged a link between infectious disease and national security. Their views are detailed in the next chapter.

CHAPTER FOUR

Defining Information Needs: Interviews with Stakeholders

Our second study objective called for assessment of the information needs of U.S. policymakers related to infectious diseases in the context of U.S. national security, and our third objective called for assessment of the adequacy of available information. Therefore, we sought input from a broad range of potential stakeholders, mostly within the federal government. This chapter describes our methods and our findings regarding stakeholder information needs, as well as the stakeholders' suggestions for enhanced information systems.

Methods

We identified each federal department with a potential interest in global infectious diseases, and within each, specific agencies or offices with specific interests in this issue. We sought to interview relatively senior policymakers or advisors in each of these organizational units, or members of their staff. We also sought the views of stakeholders outside the federal government, including representatives from the U.S. domestic public health community and the WHO. We conducted the interviews between July and October 2005.

We interviewed 53 individuals across a broad range of federal agencies and from relevant stakeholder organizations. Interviewees included 43 current and four former federal officials and six individuals from outside the federal government. Current federal staff represented the U.S. Departments of Homeland Security, Health and Human Services (HHS), Defense, State, and Agriculture (USDA); the Peace Corps; and agencies within the intelligence community. To the extent possible, we interviewed senior officials in policymaking positions or staff in their offices. As a result, nearly all the federal interviewees were within three reporting steps of a cabinet-level official or the equivalent. Nonfederal interviewees represented a state health department, the Homeland Security Institute, the U.S. Association of State and Territorial Health Officers, and the World Health Organization.[1]

---

[1] A list of all organizations included in our interviews is in Appendix A.

We asked these individuals about[2]

- the relationship between infectious diseases and national security and the role of their organizations in addressing infectious diseases
- how they use infectious disease information and the impact of their information products
- their infectious disease information needs
- their current sources of such information
- their views about open-source versus protected information
- gaps in infectious disease information
- their preferred information-delivery format
- their suggestions to improve global infectious disease information systems.

In this chapter, we summarize the views of interviewees on these questions, describing both areas of convergence and individual views that offered important insights or innovative ideas.

Results

Stakeholders Do Perceive Global Infectious Disease as a Security Threat

As described in Chapter Three, a new paradigm linking infectious disease to national security was already evolving during the 1990s, and it became more of a priority after the terror events of September and October 2001. Recent U.S. policy initiatives clearly recognize the relationship between infectious disease—both deliberate and naturally occurring threats—and national security, and seek to operationalize responses to these new threats. What is less clear is how this new paradigm is perceived across U.S. government sectors and how it has shaped the information needs of senior policymakers.

Virtually all persons we interviewed said that they believe that the global spread of infectious diseases represents a threat to U.S. national security. Some described this in narrow terms closely related to the mission of their own organization; however, the majority—including both health officials and non–health officials—described the broader-ranging impact of infectious diseases on trade, economic development, political stability, and international relations. Several elaborated on this in describing the indirect impact on jobs, productivity, and military force protection. One noted that healthy people underpin healthy economies, hence the broad benefits of investing in global health. Two individuals noted that health is a societal indicator of the public's perception of government success. Hence, less-than-successful handling of infectious disease outbreaks can undermine a population's confidence in, and ultimately the stability of, its government. Nearly all felt that both deliberate and naturally occurring diseases threaten national security. Examples of the former include smallpox, anthrax, and genetically manipulated pathogens. Examples of the latter include, among others, the broad and long-

---

[2] A list of specific interview questions is included in Appendix B.

standing impact of the HIV/AIDS pandemic; the SARS outbreak of 2002–2003; the current avian influenza H5N1 circulating in Asia, Europe, and Africa, including its potential to trigger a worldwide human influenza pandemic; and antimicrobial resistance. A number of officials across federal agencies noted that avian influenza H5N1 is their organization's current top priority. Perhaps related to this, several interviewees expressed particular concern over zoonotic diseases, i.e., human infectious diseases arising from animals. Interviewees from the USDA and one from the State Department expressed concern over plant diseases; one interviewee noted particular concern about genetically engineered pathogens, and another expressed concern about protecting the U.S. food supply.

The roles related to addressing global infectious disease spanned the breadth of the organizations represented in our interviews. The military focuses primarily on force protection; diplomats focus on humanitarian concerns, international relations, foreign policy, and the safety of Americans abroad; agriculture officials focus on protecting the domestic agriculture industry and maintaining U.S. exports; intelligence agencies are interested in the far-reaching impact of infectious diseases on political stability and U.S. national security; homeland security officials focus on protecting the United States against all security threats, including biologic threats; and health officials are responsible for protecting the public's health, both in the United States and internationally. Two individuals noted that HSPD places global infectious diseases prominently on the U.S. national security agenda. Several interviewees noted that strengthening public health infrastructures internationally is a national security priority, enabling detection and protection against both deliberate and naturally occurring infectious disease threats. These comments also encompassed veterinary health infrastructures. Several respondents also described how their own organizations and others have increasingly recognized the threats posed by global infectious diseases and hence the need to reorganize or rechannel efforts to address them.

In short, officials across government sectors perceive infectious diseases as a threat to national security and recognize both their own agency's role in addressing such threats and the larger context in which their own efforts are undertaken.

Information Supports Policy Decisions
Virtually all the federal respondents said that they need and use infectious disease information to prepare memoranda, reports, briefing papers, talking points, and strategy papers for senior-level government officials, including the President and his Cabinet secretaries. By design, most of these respondents are in policy-oriented offices and either are themselves, report directly to, or are not far removed from such senior government officials. Information on infectious disease threats has helped drive the new perception among those outside the health community of the connection between infectious disease and national security. Other respondents noted that such information is essential to relevant foreign policy decisions of the State Department, decisions by the USDA regarding the exclusion of animal and other products for import into the United States, and strategic decisions about international staffing by HHS. The State Department Bureau of Consular Affairs has used such information to prepare public announcements and travel warnings for American citizens. The State Department and Peace Corps use such information to help protect their own overseas staff, for example, the evacua-

tion of Peace Corps staff from China during the SARS outbreak. Certain information has regulatory implications, e.g., the emergence of significant drug resistance that may prompt public health announcements from the Food and Drug Administration. All respondents commented that their information products have influenced policy, including policy at the highest national and international levels. Several mentioned regular briefings to the President, Vice President, and National Security Council. Illustrative examples of infectious disease information products feeding into U.S. foreign policy include recent initiatives of the G8 and the APEC forum, international trade negotiations, and policies and actions of the most senior government officials with respect to national and foreign counterparts.

There Were More Similarities Than Differences in Information Needs Across Government Sectors

While most respondents converged around the need for timely, accurate, complete (i.e., sufficiently detailed), understandable, and actionable information related to infectious disease threats, not surprisingly, their information needs naturally focused in particular on areas directly related to the mission of their offices or agencies, or their own specific responsibilities. For example, regional focus was particularly important to individuals and offices with specific regional responsibilities; detailed health information was needed by those with specific health-related responsibilities; and non-health contextual information was most needed by the diplomatic and intelligence communities. Most respondents described needs for information about disease outbreaks that are occurring. Virtually all interviewees described needs in terms of human disease, most added the need for animal disease information, and a few mentioned an additional need for information on plant diseases. Ideally, these stakeholders would like information that reflects disease and outbreaks down to the community, rather than strictly national, level. Some recognized the shortcomings of sentinel surveillance, i.e., noncomprehensive disease surveillance from selected health service sites, emphasizing that such systems may miss important disease occurrence. Some respondents also noted the need for information on medical and health infrastructure in countries where outbreaks occur, including medical practices and government responses to the outbreaks. Several respondents described the need for information on relevant policies and decisionmaking in such countries, as well as the broader social, economic, political, and military context of disease outbreaks. They recognized that such information was unlikely to come from traditional public health sources.

Interestingly, a substantial number of health officials (both in HHS and other agencies) included broad political and economic impact among their priority information needs, and virtually all non–health officials cited traditional medical and public health information needs, e.g., clinical presentation, disease transmission patterns, disease prevention, and treatment availability and effectiveness, in helping define their own priority disease information needs. The more contextual social, economic, and political information does not lend itself to routine reporting. Also, with respect to national policies and outbreak response, several respondents noted that some countries are not timely or transparent in disease reporting and that sources other than official government reporting are important for purposes of early warning and alert. Only a few respondents described the need for anticipatory information, and did so mostly in response to direct questioning. The notable exceptions were among the intelligence community, whose information-gathering and -processing are by nature anticipatory, and within DHS, which has both anticipatory and response mandates.

Despite Similar Information Needs, Stakeholders Consult Different Information Sources

The stakeholders we interviewed described a wide range of information sources, including open-source and limited-access Web sites, official cable traffic, personal contacts with federal agency experts and federal staff overseas, and nonspecific intelligence-gathering. Most respondents use both active ("push") and passive ("pull") data-access or -delivery modes. Several subscribe to specific "push" email lists, e.g., ProMED (Program for Monitoring Emerging Diseases); U.S. Pacific Command daily alerts; or open-source tailored information alerts, such as Google Alerts™ email update service. Respondents were generally familiar with a larger number of Web sites than they actually used. Among the most frequently consulted open Web sites, consulted largely on a "pull" basis, are those of the CDC and the WHO. Well-regarded password-protected or subscription-based Web sites are the CDC's Epi-X (Epidemic Information Exchange), the Foreign Broadcast Information Service, and GPHIN. Respondents also reported consulting directly with experts within their own departments, federal staff in other departments, and experts outside the U.S. government. Some interviewees (e.g., those in different parts of the State Department) rely on colleagues to send them information when and as appropriate. Respondents who drew upon personal contacts for key information valued this type of information source greatly, since direct discussion yields the timely and tailored information they need.

Classification of Information Is Important but Creates Some Obstacles

Respondents across all government agencies recognize the importance of both open-source and protected information, including information related to infectious diseases. However, some agencies (e.g., the Peace Corps and HHS) noted their sensitivity to international perceptions that their staff may have links to the intelligence community, and they felt that such perceptions jeopardize their good standing with key national counterparts and, hence, limit their ability to operate effectively. Information is classified to protect sources and methods. Sensitive content relates to potential U.S. vulnerabilities, including bioterrorism, military movements, new medical countermeasures under development (e.g., intellectual property protection), information needed for diplomatic leverage, and information that is politically sensitive to the United States. Several respondents commented that some unclassified information arrives via classified channels, e.g., reporting cables with both classified and unclassified sections, and as a result may be unnecessarily inaccessible to a broader range of government officials who do not have the necessary clearances. A number of respondents cited inadequate security clearances as an impediment to optimal information-sharing. For example, some respondents from the intelligence community said that HHS staff do not necessarily have the full range of security clearances they probably need. Also, the domestic public health establishment typically and systematically lacks security clearances that would facilitate their emergency preparedness planning.

Stakeholders' Information Needs Are Not Fully Met by Their Current Sources

Respondents noted many gaps related to global infectious disease information. Many respondents noted the current ad hoc nature of information, i.e., a lack of systematic inputs and outputs. Many commented on the glut of available information and the resulting need for information management processes to enhance delivery, presentation, and efficient data use. One respondent commented, "There is never enough information when you need it, but otherwise there is too much information." According to another respondent, the need is not necessarily for more information, but for the right information that is accessible in a timely fashion through a convenient delivery mechanism. Several respondents commented on the gap in relevant international agriculture-sector disease data. One noted that some information, e.g., detailed animal disease surveillance data, is not collected in some countries and hence is simply not available. This particular gap can be due to poor infrastructure and/or lack of appropriate incentives to report animal disease.

The majority of respondents noted that agencies across the federal government need the same basic information, and that several agencies have important information, but that information is not widely shared. For example, one office reported that its secretary, a major stakeholder, had to contact the director of national intelligence to ask for information after learning that the President was being briefed on a strategic global infectious disease issue without direct input from his department. Other shortcomings in currently available information include inadequate timeliness, accuracy, completeness, and larger contextual analysis. Gaps relate to both "signals intelligence" (e.g., communications about local disease outbreaks or animal die-offs) and "human intelligence" (e.g., information based on direct observation or personal contacts). Several respondents commented that what is lacking is a resource to coordinate and consolidate public health and other information and share useful, common analytic products with stakeholders across government.

Questions about specific disease scenarios (i.e., SARS, avian influenza, the next—as yet unknown—emerging disease, or any other infectious disease threat of particular concern) yielded additional insights. For example, respondents from several government agencies noted that overseas-based U.S. federal staff, including their own staff, are the "eyes and ears on the ground" to help identify and sort out early information about emerging outbreaks. Several respondents commented that infectious disease problems require new sources and types of "public health intelligence" and that more non-U.S. sources are needed. One official in a regulatory agency would like information on domestic surge capacity needs, particularly as related to the medical supplies and equipment his agency regulates.

Preferences Vary for Information-Delivery Format and Methods

Nearly all respondents commented on the overwhelming amount of information and the need for efficiency in obtaining desired information. Many respondents draw upon both "push" and "pull" sources of information. Preferences for the former include selected or customizable email alerts, i.e., providing information limited to their specific topical, regional, or other defined interests. Virtually no respondent expressed a desire for broad, frequent, nonselective "push" information. A notable exception was one official who reported directly to a cabinet secretary and commented that he prefers "push" approaches and would like to know more rather than less because information that is too filtered is useless, and one risks missing early clues to a subsequent significant threat. Currently, "push" information is based largely on unofficial reporting, including the media, rather than official—and more traditional—government reporting. Preferred "pull" information is mostly from Web sites, notably those of the CDC and WHO, and direct consultation with technical experts or overseas staff.

Not surprisingly, the preferred format and presentation of information varied by both agency and the level of the individual within her or his agency. For example, those higher in the federal structure tended to prefer filtered or processed information presented as concise analysis products, including daily or weekly summaries of a single disease or a handful of key diseases. Those responsible for preparing briefings and papers for senior officials need more detailed information, including basic disease information and reports on the status of an ongoing outbreak, preferably based on validated case reports. Respondents outside the health sector commented on the need for information to be presented in a way that they as non–health policymakers can readily understand and use, including contextual political and economic information and implications.

Stakeholders Suggested Areas for Improvement

Virtually all respondents offered suggestions and insights for improving global infectious disease information. They generally framed their suggestions to address both bioterrorism and naturally occurring disease threats, easing what some viewed as disproportionate attention to deliberate threats at the expense of more likely threat scenarios. A common suggestion was for improved detection capacity and timeliness and transparency of disease reporting by foreign governments. However, these are not necessarily within the direct purview of the United States. At least two respondents called upon the United States to invest more in the disease surveillance activities of foreign governments. This would serve the dual purpose of helping to strengthen foreign public health infrastructures for the collective good and providing opportunities for more U.S. "eyes and ears on the ground" working in mutually trusting relationships with their national counterparts, making them potentially privy to early disease outbreak information. One State Department official also described his plans for taking fuller advantage of embassy staff and the U.S. business community in foreign countries through better briefings to sensitize them about possible disease threats and encourage them to report back. In contrast, two individuals from the intelligence community commented that the current era of global communications limits the need for additional U.S. personnel in the field. Several respondents commented on the need for different government agencies to understand and interact more fruitfully with one another. One interviewee noted that there might not be sufficient focus on health at the highest levels in the U.S. government security apparatus, which would be affirmatively demonstrated by the appointment of a dedicated health and medical expert to the National Security Council.

Most current federal employees we interviewed offered one or more specific suggestions for a centralized, time-sensitive (i.e., reliably current), integrated, coordinated U.S. government–wide system. Only one office, interviewed after a full month of completed interviews (approximately 25 percent of the total number of interviews), explicitly mentioned the new National Biosurveillance Integration System, coordinated by the Department of Homeland

Security (see Chapter Three for further details on NBIS). Even when those interviewed subsequently were directly queried, very few were aware of NBIS. Their suggestions were therefore largely independent of, but highly consistent with, the intended features of NBIS. The suggestions of different respondents included a system with the following attributes to collect and disseminate information on the occurrence of and risks for infectious disease threats: (1) top-down creation of a better environment for information-sharing, which in turn would help optimize agency budgets and break down agency "silos" to collect and share information most efficiently; (2) a single integrated system with "robust capabilities" that would provide "science-based actionable information" to the full range of stakeholders, in the format most appropriate for each; (3) 24/7 access to experts, as needed, to anticipate or respond to specific threats; (4) a central data repository for "pull" access, as needed, including links to more detailed information for those interested; (5) use of data-mining and other methods for active information collection; (6) an expanded collection that encompasses a broader range of pathogen hosts (i.e., animal and plant diseases) and a broader range of foreign language sources; (7) systematic data filtering to help distinguish signal from noise; (8) reconciliation of conflicting information from different sources, e.g., those about a specific disease or outbreak; (9) information system interoperability; and (10) avoidance of duplication of efforts. Several respondents commented that they would welcome a multilateral or philanthropic initiative to collect, integrate, coordinate, and actively disseminate open-source information on infectious disease threats worldwide. One respondent further suggested a strong "marketing" initiative to educate federal stakeholders regarding sources of available infectious disease information, including intervention measures.

Summary

There is now an impressively broad range of government stakeholders interested in information on worldwide infectious disease threats. As noted in Chapter Three, health professionals increasingly recognize the broader social, economic, and political impact of these diseases, and officials in other sectors and agencies increasingly appreciate the transition of infectious diseases and public health into the realm of high politics.[3] As presented in this chapter, stakeholders across government sectors described their need for information that is both directly related to their own agency's responsibilities and also beyond their direct areas of action, e.g., beyond more technical disease information for security and diplomatic officials and broader economic and political information for health officials.

In beginning to address our third research question about the adequacy of current information, the majority of federal officials we interviewed called for better efficiency and coordination of information collection, processing, and dissemination across the federal government

---

[3] A more detailed discussion of the ascendance of health from "low politics" to "high politics" can be found in Lee, Buse, and Fustukian (2002), which also references a definition of "high politics": "First, in foreign policy analysis, it is used as a collective expression for certain issue areas of crucial importance" (citing Evans and Newnham, 1992).

and to other stakeholders as possible, including U.S. state and local and foreign governments, and multilateral organizations engaged in global infectious disease prevention and control. In the next chapter, we further address this question.

CHAPTER FIVE

Assessing the Adequacy of Current Information: A Survey of Online Sources

Our third research question asks about the adequacy of currently available information related to global infectious disease. The preceding chapter summarized the views of stakeholders regarding current information sources and ideas for improvements. In this chapter, we describe a more systematic assessment of currently available information.

We compiled and assessed Internet-based ("online") sources of information relevant to infectious diseases globally (see Appendix C for the complete list and brief descriptions of the sources we assessed). Online information sources are added or changed frequently. Therefore, while not purporting to have captured all such sources, we encompassed a number and range of online sources that is sufficient to both assess the nature of current online information and serve as a potentially useful resource for U.S. policymakers. A comprehensive analysis of the content or quality of these sources was beyond the scope of this project. This chapter describes our methods and the detailed descriptive analyses of the key characteristics of these sources, based on our survey.

Methods

We identified potential online sources through four mechanisms: (1) online searches using terms such as "disease surveillance," "infectious disease network," "infectious disease alert," "disease surveillance bulletin," and "ministry of health"; (2) a review of pertinent published literature; (3) a review of a limited list of compiled online sources from a separate, unpublished RAND project that sought approximately similar online sources; and (4) suggestions from our interviewees. The sources we compiled focused predominately on human diseases but also included animal and plant diseases relevant to human health. We reviewed all potential online sources to ascertain accessibility and content directly relevant to the public health aspects of infectious diseases or useful in support of disease control. We retained sources that were both accessible (or could be described based on publicly available information online or in the literature, if the sources were accessible only via authorization or subscription) and that we considered sufficiently relevant, as described below. We extracted key information on each source and created a standardized database describing their features to enable analysis and to facilitate searches based on selected features. We captured the following information, when available, for each source:

- general information
  - name
  - sponsor: name of organization
  - sponsor category: multilateral (global, regional), national (U.S. national, state, foreign), nongovernmental organization (NGO), professional/academic, commercial
  - Web address
  - brief description
  - geographic reach (global, regional—with named region, national—with named country, subnational—with name of local district (e.g., U.S. state)
  - primary purpose: surveillance (general), surveillance (early warning), surveillance bulletin, terrorism, reference or research resources, others
  - data content
  - specific disease, if any (otherwise, "various")

- data input
  - host species (human, animal, and/or plant)
  - data source(s)
  - active or passive data collection
  - voluntary or mandatory data reporting
  - standardized or non-standardized data reporting
  - cases or outbreaks
  - disease-specific or symptom or syndrome-based
  - frequency of reporting
  - data analysis process
  - limitations in access to the source (e.g., password-protected, subscription-only)
  - limitations in data quality (e.g., outdated, missing information; low specificity; foreign language)
  - sdditional notes, if any

- data output
  - active or passive dissemination
  - audience
  - frequency or timeliness of dissemination
  - standardized or nonstandardized data format
  - reporting based on individual cases or outbreaks
  - type of information outputs
  - value or veracity, i.e., if and how data are verified before dissemination.

Following completion of the database, we distributed it on a test basis to interviewees who had expressed an interest in such a tool. We also tabulated the number of sources according to the various characteristics described above.

Results

The remainder of this chapter summarizes key characteristics of these online sources. It is organized into the following sections: accessibility of information; organizational sponsorship; primary purpose, with further discussion of general and early warning surveillance sources; human and nonhuman disease sources; active and passive information collection; and information dissemination.

Most Online Sources Have Unrestricted Access

As shown in Figure 5.1, nearly two-thirds of all sources (62 percent, 144 sources) are accessible without limitation, 29 percent (68 sources) require authorization,[1] and 9 percent (22 sources) require either paid or solicited subscription.[2] Of the 144 unrestricted-access sources, slightly over half (79 sources, or 55 percent) function primarily for surveillance purposes, and one-quarter are reference sources (36 sources, 25 percent). The remaining open-access sources have research (10 sources, 7 percent) or other primary functions (19 sources, 13 percent). The sponsors of open-access sources cover a broad range, including U.S. agencies at both the national and state levels (42 sources, 29 percent), multilateral organizations at both global (20 sources, 14 percent) and regional (11 sources, 8 percent) levels, foreign countries (39 sources, 27 percent), professional/academic organizations (20 sources, 14 percent), and commercial (six sources, 4 percent) and nongovernmental organizations (six sources, 4 percent). Open-access sites include global (45 sources, 32 percent), regional (15 sources, 10 percent), or national information, including U.S. (36 sources, 25 percent) or foreign (48 sources, 33 percent) national. Most of them provide information on a passive, or "pull" basis rather than pushing information out to users.

Three-fourths of the 68 sources requiring authorized access, i.e., not fully open sources, focus on surveillance: general surveillance (30 sources, 45 percent), early warning surveillance (11 sources, 16 percent), or surveillance bulletins (10 sources, 15 percent). The remaining 24 percent of these sources is evenly distributed across other primary functions (between two and four sources in each category). Nearly two-thirds of the sources that require authorized access are from U.S national or state sponsors (43 sources, 63 percent); just over 10 percent (seven sources) are sponsored by professional or academic organizations; and the remaining sources are sponsored by multilateral organizations (eight sources, 12 percent), foreign countries (six sources, 9 percent), commercial entities (three sources, 4 percent), or NGOs (one source, 2 percent).

---

[1] Authorization is defined here as access obtained through permission granted by the source host, such as ministries of health surveillance systems that participate in WHO global surveillance programs.

[2] Paid subscription refers to access through a purchased membership to a Web-based service, whereas solicited refers to access granted upon request or registration to a notification list.

Figure 5.1
Accessibility of Online Sources

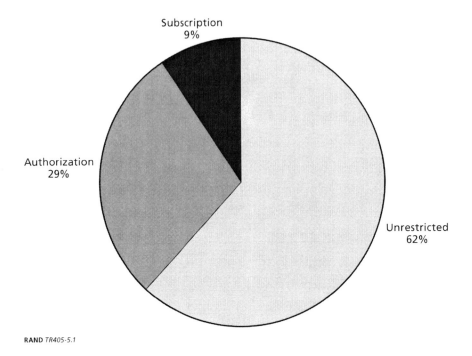

RAND *TR405-5.1*

The U.S. federal government sponsors 39 of the sources that require authorization for access (the remaining four U.S. government sources are from U.S. state agencies):

- Department of Defense (18 sources)
- Department of Health and Human Services, Centers for Disease Control and Prevention (16 sources)
- Department of Energy (two sources)
- U.S. Department of Agriculture (one source)
- Department of Veterans Affairs (one source)
- Central Intelligence Agency (one source).

The 22 sources (9 percent) requiring a subscription serve various purposes, including reference (seven sources, 32 percent), antiterrorism (seven sources, 32 percent), surveillance (five sources, 23 percent), or other purposes (three sources, 14 percent). Slightly more than three-fourths of subscription-based sources (17 sources, 77 percent) are sponsored by commercial organizations, with professional and academic organizations sponsoring three (14 percent) and foreign governments sponsoring two (9 percent) sources. Subscription-based sources focus primarily on U.S. national (13 sources, 59 percent) or global (eight sources, 36 percent) information.

Online Sources Reflect a Broad Range of Organizational Sponsors

Partly because of the focus of our search and the type of information we sought, the 234 online sources come largely from government sponsors (see Figure 5.2). These included 36 percent (85 sources) from U.S. government agencies at the federal and state levels, e.g., from HHS (several from CDC), DoD, USDA, DHS, and others. Twenty percent of sources (47) are from foreign governments, and a combined 16 percent are from global (24 sources, 10 percent) and regional (15 sources, 6 percent) multilateral organizations, such as the WHO, the Pan American Health Organization (PAHO), the Office International des Epizoöties (World Animal Health Organization) (OIE), and the Food and Agriculture Organization of the United Nations (FAO). The remaining sources are sponsored by professional or academic, commercial, or non-governmental organizations.

Nearly one-third of all sources (76 sources, 32 percent) are global in coverage; 21 sources (9 percent) focus on regional coverage; and the remainder focus on national coverage, including U.S. national or subnational (81 sources, 35 percent) and foreign national (56 sources, 24 percent).[3] The foreign national and regional sources collectively span the globe, including Europe (33 sources), Asia and the Pacific (24 sources), the Americas (11 sources), Africa (5 sources), and the Middle East (4 sources).

Figure 5.2
Organizational Sponsors of Online Sources

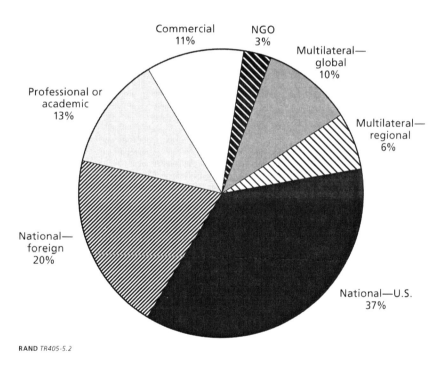

RAND *TR405-5.2*

---

[3] Foreign national, as used in this and subsequent sections, refers to non-U.S. countries.

Over Half the 234 Sources Focus on Surveillance, Including Early Warning

Our study focused in particular on information related to infectious disease surveillance and public health. Over half our online sources related to disease surveillance, including 98 general surveillance (42 percent), 23 surveillance bulletins (10 percent), and 14 surveillance early warning (6 percent). (See Figure 5.3.)

Surveillance systems collect and monitor information to identify disease trends or outbreaks. Early warning surveillance plays a more active role in acquiring and disseminating timely (especially daily or near–real-time) information on specific diseases or less specific indicators and warnings, often reflecting early rumors rather than confirmed diagnoses, but intending to serve the purpose of timely alert to a potential problem.[4] Surveillance bulletins function as official information dissemination routes and information archives for surveillance data and tend to be sites closely linked to actual surveillance systems. Examples of these

Figure 5.3
Primary Purpose of Online Sources

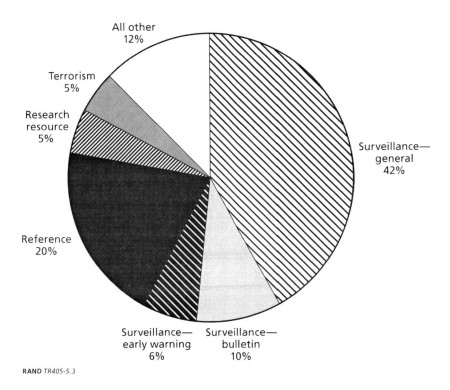

RAND *TR405-5.3*

---

[4] While early warning surveillance systems, especially syndromic surveillance (reports of disease diagnosed clinically without laboratory confirmation), can be highly sensitive in detecting disease events, but they often suffer from low specificity. This trade-off can increase the proportion of false positives compared with other surveillance systems. Moreover, attribution of an epidemic to the incorrect disease can trigger inappropriate interventions. Verification through investigation and definitive diagnosis (e.g., as the WHO does through its GOARN program) can offset this problem and has proven extraordinarily useful. Additionally, most early warning systems in the United States have provided early detection of mild to moderately severe outbreaks but not outbreaks of severe disease.

sources include the CDC *Morbidity and Mortality Weekly Report*, the WHO *Weekly Epidemiological Report*, and *Eurosurveillance* bulletins (weekly, monthly, and quarterly surveillance summaries on diseases in the European region).

Table 5.1 compares the characteristics of sources serving general surveillance and early warning surveillance functions. Most (87 of 98 sources, 89 percent) of the general surveillance sources in our database focus on human disease information, including 73 sources (74 percent) that focus exclusively on human diseases and 14 sources (14 percent) that also include animal and/or plant disease; the remaining general surveillance sources (11 sources, 11 percent) address animal diseases only.

We were particularly interested in the 14 sources (6 percent) that provide early warning information. Most of them (nine) are U.S. government sources addressing various diseases. All 14 address human disease, including one that also addresses animal and plant diseases. Half (seven) of the sources have largely U.S. national reach, five have global reach, and one each is specific to a country (Pakistan) or a region (Southeast Asia). Not surprisingly, most of these early warning sources employ active data collection (eight of 14 sources) and active dissemination (seven of 14), with two-thirds (nine of 14) disseminating information daily or on a near–real-time basis. In contrast, data collection and dissemination from general surveillance sources are more likely through passive methods, and dissemination frequency is more variable, from daily or near–real-time (11 percent) to frequencies ranging from weekly to annual (42 percent), or ad hoc dissemination (28 percent).

Beyond the largest group of online sources focusing on surveillance, 47 primarily serve reference purposes (20 percent). Reference sources contain a wide range of information, such as a virologic database, a directory of surveillance systems, a searchable database of documented global disease outbreaks, and a virtual information center that posts disease announcements.

Twelve sources (5 percent) are categorized as research resources and serve as data centers or online archives of reports, or contain analytic tools intended for open use by researchers. Among the remaining sources, 11 (5 percent) primarily serve antiterrorism purposes, and a small handful each serve laboratory, networking, communications, or other primary purposes.

The majority of sources focus exclusively on specific diseases (141 sources, 60 percent), rather than on syndromes (13 sources, 6 percent).[5] Some (27 sources, 12 percent) include information on both diseases and syndromes; this information is unknown or not applicable for the remaining sources (53 sources, 23 percent). Most sources (146, 62 percent) include information on a broad range of infectious diseases. Several sources address a defined set of diseases or pathogens, and others are dedicated sources, focusing on a single pathogen, disease, or issue (e.g., influenza, tuberculosis, gonorrhea, measles, antimicrobial resistance, biothreat agents).

---

[5] A *syndrome* is the concurrence of several symptoms that collectively indicate a type of illness but not a specific disease diagnosis.

Table 5.1
General Surveillance and Early Warning Surveillance Online Sources

Characteristic	General Surveillance Sources		Early Warning Surveillance Sources	
	N	%	N	%
Total	98	100	14	100
Sponsor category				
Multilateral—global	11	11	0	0
Multilateral—regional	8	8	0	0
National—U.S.	36	37	9	64
National—U.S. state	3	3	0	0
National—non-U.S.	25	26	2	14
Academic/professional	8	8	3	22
Commercial	5	5	0	0
NGO	2	2	0	0
Geographic coverage				
National—U.S.	34	35	7	50
National—non-U.S.	34	35	1	7
Global	18	18	5	36
Regional	12	12	1	7
Disease host				
Human	74	75	13	93
Animal and human	13	13	0	0
Animal	11	11	0	0
Animal, human, and plant	1	1	1	7
Frequency of information dissemination				
Ad hoc	28	28	4	29
Annual	16	16	0	0
Weekly to biannually	26	26	1	7
Daily or near real-time	11	11	9	64
Unknown	18	18	0	0

NOTE: The data in this table reflect only the 112 general and early warning surveillance sources; the remaining 122 sources do not address these areas.

Sources Include Information on Diseases in Humans, Animals, and Plants

Because of the nature of our search and the focus of this study, most of the online sources we compiled address human diseases. However, the evolving nature of emerging diseases (described in Chapter Two) and the threat of terrorism are reflected in the substantial number of online sources that include information on animal or plant diseases. As shown in Figure 5.4, a total of 87 percent of sources (205 sources) address human diseases, 24 percent (57 sources) address animal diseases, and 4–5 percent (11 sources) address plant diseases. However, many sources include combinations of the three.

Nearly all the 57 sources with information on animal diseases have unrestricted access (50 sources, 88 percent). The 57 sources are sponsored mostly by U.S. government agencies at the national or state level (16 sources, 28 percent), multilateral organizations (13 sources, 23 percent), foreign governments (12 sources, 21 percent), and professional or academic organizations (11 sources, 19 percent). These sources predominantly serve surveillance (34 sources, 60 percent) or reference (16 sources, 28 percent) purposes. Similarly, most of the 11 sources with information on plant diseases have unrestricted access (eight sources, 73 percent), but they are more evenly distributed across types of sponsoring organizations and serve a wider range of purposes, particularly reference or research (each, 3 sources, 27 percent).

Figure 5.4
Sources Addressing Human, Animal, and Plant Diseases

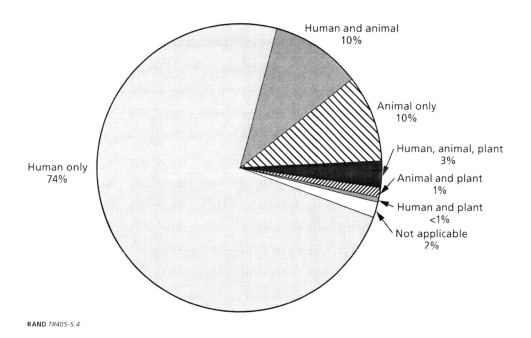

RAND *TR405-5.4*

Nearly One-Third of Our Sources Use Active Information Collection Methods

A key element used to characterize online sources of disease information is the way in which the information presented by sources is collected. The method of information collection is an important consideration in the interpretation, application, and ultimate use of information by policymakers. Passive data collection, which is typically used in traditional disease surveillance, denotes an approach in which disease information reaches sponsors—usually government authorities and health departments—through a voluntary or mandatory reporting system that includes primary data sources, such as clinical facilities and laboratories. In contrast, active data collection denotes a system in which sponsors seek out disease information, e.g., through site visits, medical records reviews, or surveys. Active data collection processes are particularly important in the context of surveillance—especially early warning surveillance—and emerging infections as a way to closely monitor, detect, and respond to disease occurrence in a timely fashion. The approach to the collection of health information depends largely on the objectives and capabilities of sponsor organizations.

We examined our online sources to determine their approach to data collection. Overall, 26 percent of sources (61 sources) use active methods only, 63 percent (146 sources) use passive methods only, and 5 percent (12 sources) use both active and passive methods; this information is unknown or not applicable for 6 percent of sources (15 sources) (see Figure 5.5).[6] Thus,

Figure 5.5
Information Collection Methods of Online Sources

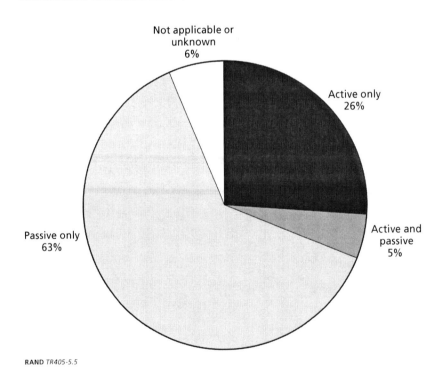

RAND *TR405-5.5*

---

6   Some sources do not collect information but instead serve other purposes, such as reference or research support.

31 percent of sources use active data collection and 69 percent use passive data collection, with 12 sources using a combination of methods included in both categories.

While most online sources reflect passive information collection, we were particularly interested in those that obtain data through active methods (73 sources, 31 percent overall; 61 sources, 26 percent using active methods only). As shown in Table 5.2, active data collection methods are more common than passive methods among sources that serve antiterrorism, networking, communication, and early warning surveillance purposes. Multilateral regional

Table 5.2
Characteristics of Sources Using Active or Passive Information Collection

Characteristic	Active Sources		Passive Sources	
	N	%	N	%
Total	73	100	158	100
Primary purpose				
General surveillance	25	25	79	80
Surveillance bulletin	6	26	17	74
Early warning surveillance	8	57	7	50
Reference	11	23	32	68
Research resource site	4	33	7	58
Terrorism	7	64	1	9
Networking	4	67	2	33
Communication	3	100	0	0
Laboratory	0	0	2	100
Other early warning acts	2	67	0	0
Other	3	20	12	80
Sponsor category				
Multilateral—global	6	25	19	79
Multilateral—regional	7	47	9	60
National—U.S.	22	28	55	70
National—U.S. state	2	29	5	71
National—non-U.S.	15	31	34	71
Academic/professional	8	28	20	69
Commercial	11	42	12	46
NGO	2	29	5	71

Table 5.2—Continued

Characteristic	Active Sources		Passive Sources	
	N	%	N	%
Geographic coverage				
Global	19	25	54	71
National—U.S.	30	41	39	53
National—non-U.S.	17	30	51	91
Regional	7	33	15	71
Disease host				
Animal	6	26	17	74
Human	50	29	118	68
Animal and human	9	38	17	71
Animal and plant	0	0	3	100
Animal, human, and plant	6	86	2	29
Not applicable	2	67	1	33
Standardization				
Standardized	21	32	45	69
Semi-standardized	27	33	56	68
Not standardized	19	28	46	68
Mixed	3	100	2	67
Unknown	3	30	4	40
Not applicable	0	0	6	86

NOTE: The data columns reflect *any* active or passive collection. Twelve sources use both methods and are counted in both categories.

organizations and commercial sponsors were more likely than others to use active data collection methods. Finally, sources with comprehensive information on human, animal, and plant diseases were more likely to use active information collection than were sources with information limited to human or animal diseases only.

About One-Third of Sources Actively Disseminate Their Data Output

Nearly one-third of online sources (76 sources, 32 percent) use active or "push" data dissemination; the remainder use passive or "pull" dissemination. Active dissemination takes the form of government notification to health providers regarding disease updates, email alerts and other communications to relevant authorities, and public announcements by health departments. Passive or "pull" dissemination in the context of these online sources means that information is available for users to consult, but users are not actively notified of such information. Sources with information collected through active means are more likely to disseminate their output actively (48 percent), compared with active dissemination from sources using passive data collection methods (23 percent, chi-square = 15.348, df = 1, p = 0.00009). Sources that actively "push" their data output also disseminate information more frequently than do sources that rely mostly on passive "pull" dissemination: Forty percent of the former, but only 7 percent of the latter, update or disseminate their data on a daily or near–real-time basis.

Summary

In this chapter, we described an array of online infectious disease information sources that could be used by a range of technical experts and policy staff to inform policy decisions. These sources vary according to their accessibility, organizational sponsors, primary purposes, disease hosts, information collection methods, timeliness of data collection and output, and other characteristics. We undertook this compilation of sources because our literature review indicated that there were potentially many information sources available but few, if any, sources that compile, analyze, and distribute the large amount of available information in a comprehensive and useful manner. Early interviews during this study indicated that identifying useful and relevant sources of information among the many sources available is a significant challenge, further prompting the analysis in this chapter. The database we compiled was not intended to result in an authoritative compendium of online sources; it cannot be exhaustive, since the population of online sources changes continuously. The database was intended primarily to allow for the above descriptive analysis, to inform response to our third research question regarding the adequacy of current information. However, several U.S. government stakeholders we interviewed expressed considerable interest in the database, and we have given it to them for their use. In addition, the online sources from our database could be relevant to DHS as it further develops NBIS, i.e., by adding our sources to the large number of sources from which NBIS currently draws its information. Our sources likewise span a wide range of infectious disease information, from comprehensive to disease-specific, from human to animal and plant diseases, from domestic to foreign, and from surveillance to widely ranging support information related to infectious diseases.

CHAPTER SIX

Synthesis, Conclusions, and Recommendations

Synthesis

As described throughout this report, a key theme regarding infectious diseases over the past century, and likely into the future, is change. Some changes present challenges, while others present opportunities. The world is being challenged by a resurgence of infectious disease mortality; the emergence and rapid spread of new diseases, including zoonotic diseases and diseases resistant to antimicrobial drugs; and the broad impact of infectious diseases on trade, security, and economic development. Opportunities arise from new perspectives, new stakeholders, new technologies, and new approaches to disease detection and control. The following discussion synthesizes challenges, opportunities, and new initiatives related to global infectious diseases, focusing on transformations in disease evolution, the way U.S. policymakers can think about and respond to infectious disease challenges around the world, and implications for the future. The chapter then concludes with our responses to the three original questions addressed in this study and our recommendations for further action.

New Diseases with Global Distribution

Emerging and reemerging infectious diseases have posed numerous challenges over recent decades. Factors associated with the emergence and spread of these diseases include ecological changes, human demographics and behavior, international travel and trade, changes in land use, inadequacy and deterioration of public health infrastructures worldwide, microbial adaptation and change, misuse of antimicrobial drugs, and others. The CDC and the Committee on International Science, Engineering, and Technology (CISET) reported 30 examples of pathogens that emerged or reemerged between 1973 and 1995 (CDC, 1998; CISET, 1995). More recent examples include SARS and avian influenza H5N1. These have captured attention because of their spread across countries, illustrating yet again that diseases know no borders in this age of globalization, and an infectious disease threat anywhere in the world can become a threat everywhere.

New Populations of Interest: Diseases in Animals

Zoonotic diseases represent approximately three-fourths of newly emerged and reemerged infectious diseases in recent decades. As the current avian influenza H5N1 outbreaks illustrate, this means that disease surveillance and control must extend beyond the human population into the animal population. This requires veterinary health infrastructures as well as those for human public health. While human public health infrastructures may range in strength across different countries, animal health infrastructures are often lacking altogether.

New Perspectives

Recent high-profile diseases such as SARS and avian influenza have served to underscore the relatively new view of some infectious diseases as a threat to national security. They have captured attention through their broad impact not only on health but also on international trade, security, and national economies. During the 1990s, economists and political scientists increasingly considered HIV/AIDS a broad threat to economic development, national stability, and national security. For example, the real or perceived decimation of foreign militaries by HIV and the loss of productive workers across all economic sectors undermine economic and social development and threaten political stability. The more recent outbreak of SARS and the almost-certain prospect of a human influenza pandemic, whether or not it arises from the currently circulating H5N1 avian influenza strain, have raised heightened concern because of their potential for even more rapid and extensive spread. Further, the current avian influenza outbreaks in Asia and eastern Europe are a constant reminder of the links between the public health sector and the agriculture, trade, tourism, economic, and political sectors, and thus not only the collective impact of such diseases but also the opportunity for collective, i.e., stronger, actions to combat them.

New Range of Stakeholders Interested in Global Infectious Diseases

These new perspectives on infectious diseases in the age of globalization have given rise to a broader range of stakeholders, i.e., leaders not just from the health sector but also from the agriculture, trade, tourism, economic, foreign affairs, security, and political sectors. This is our reason for interviewing a broad range of stakeholders with the objective of soliciting views regarding current information needs of U.S. policymakers (see Chapter Four). As a result of the broader range of stakeholders now concerned with infectious disease, leadership on these "health" issues has extended into new domains, resulting in initiatives from such groups as the UN General Assembly, the G8, the APEC forum, the Association of Southeast Asian Nations (ASEAN), and others. Shared leadership presents both the significant opportunities and the broad challenges of working effectively across different sectors that may have different cultures, incentives, and methods and that typically do not interact directly with one another.

New Active Information-Gathering Approaches

Traditionally, infectious disease surveillance information has come from passive reporting of clinical or laboratory data to government officials, often with significant delay. Active data collection approaches can range from labor-intensive human outreach to obtain clinical or laboratory data to automated active data collection methods. GPHIN is just one example of automated data collection that serves an important surveillance and early warning function. It employs data-mining techniques to actively search worldwide media sources in various languages; data are quickly analyzed in Canada and then sent to the WHO for verification with affected countries. The U.S. government's new biosurveillance system, NBIS, is intended to employ active and extensive data-mining approaches to provide early warning signals relevant to infectious diseases worldwide. These are both promising early warning systems to improve sensitivity and timeliness of disease alerts.

New Sources of Information

Our study, including the literature review, interviews with a broad range of government officials, and the compilation of online data sources, has supported the hypothesis that governments are no longer the sole, or perhaps even the most reliable, sources of information on infectious diseases. NGOs (e.g., the Global Disaster Information Network), the media (e.g., sources actively accessed via GPHIN), and Internet discussion groups (e.g., ProMED) are increasingly providing critical early warning of outbreaks. As noted in Chapter Two, the WHO has acknowledged that a significant proportion of confirmed outbreaks are first reported by such sources, rather than by affected governments. Approximately one-fourth of the 234 online sources we compiled were sponsored by NGOs, professional or academic institutions, or commercial sources; moreover, even some government-sponsored sources (e.g., GPHIN, NBIS) draw information from media sources rather than from official government reports.

New Disease Indicators

Traditional disease reporting has been based on government notification of clinical diagnoses, especially hospital inpatients or clinic outpatients, or laboratory testing. However, less traditional indicators of disease cases and outbreaks offer promise as well and are being implemented through new initiatives. For example, retail sales of over-the-counter medicines, the tracking of which is part of the U.S. BioSense initiative, can indicate localized surges in demand for treatments for respiratory and diarrheal diseases and, hence, serve as a community indicator of disease occurrence. School absenteeism has been used in the past as a potential early warning proxy for community spread of disease, such as influenza-like illness or other respiratory disease; however, this approach has been discontinued. These are just two examples of indicators that complement the more traditional disease indicators and hence may offer added value in terms of comprehensiveness (because they do not rely strictly on persons seeking clinical care) and potentially timeliness (such reports may come earlier than government notification through official surveillance reporting). It will be important to consider comparably innovative indicators for animal and plant infections that have the potential for spread to humans.

New Ways of Reporting

Local, national, and international media increasingly report on infectious disease occurrences. SARS and avian influenza H5N1 are recent examples. The media serve to provide timely information to a broader audience (i.e., the general public) than the more traditional information that is channeled almost exclusively through government sources. GPHIN and NBIS capitalize upon active data-mining techniques to capture such information. Additionally, the Internet has facilitated a revolution in real-time information dissemination. Infectious disease information is reported through a number of active and passive mechanisms. Distribution lists, such as ProMED, APEC Emerging Infections Network (EINet), and others, push general information to users; Google Alerts and other sources actively provide more tailored information based on user requests. The stakeholders we interviewed expressed strong wishes for tailored information that meets their needs without being overwhelming.

New Types of Analysis and Presentation

With the growing breadth of infections across host species and the accompanying growing interest in government sectors, it has become increasingly important to consider ways to integrate information from individual sources and make it useful and usable by all relevant stakeholders. This was a clear message from the stakeholders we interviewed. Thus, public health and veterinary health data must be integrated with more contextual and analytic information from the security, foreign affairs, and intelligence sectors. Further, information must be presented in a way that is understandable, and preferably actionable, even to non–health experts and non-policymakers. Disease information presentation can be in the form of numbers, tables, or maps, and it may be more fully analyzed in terms of context and broader implications. The USDA's Center for Emerging Issues worksheets provide a good example of more complete analysis and reporting of infectious disease issues—in this case, those that are relevant to the agriculture sector.

New Policy Initiatives

Finally, the United States has established a number of recent high-level policy initiatives to operationalize responses to infectious disease threats within the context of national security. All of these either represent or depend upon information related to infectious diseases. These initiatives are unprecedented in two regards: They make clear the connection between infectious disease and security, and they involve U.S. presidential leadership on what might otherwise be considered simply health issues. A number are domestically oriented initiatives addressing bioterrorism threats, stemming mostly from the 2004 HSPD-10/NSPD-33. However, the majority are internationally oriented bilateral and multilateral initiatives. These include a 1996 Presidential Decision Directive to operationalize the U.S. global EID strategy (see White House 1996b); U.S. leadership to bring the first health issue (HIV/AIDS) to the UN Security Council (2000); U.S. leadership in the 2001 establishment of the Global Fund to Fight AIDS, Tuberculosis and Malaria; the President's 2002 Emergency Plan for AIDS Relief; the APEC Health Security Initiative (2003); and the 2005 International Partnership on Avian and Pandemic Influenza. In addition, planning for a nationwide U.S. response to pandemic influenza is under way at the highest levels of government, as demonstrated by President Bush's release of the *National Strategy for Pandemic Influenza* and the *HHS Pandemic Influenza Plan*.[1] The number and high political profile of these recent initiatives clearly signals the escalation of infectious disease threats into the realm of high politics and makes it all the more important for stakeholders across government sectors to have the information they need to implement these initiatives.

---

[1] White House (2005) and U.S. Department of Health and Human Services (2005), respectively. Both documents are also available through http://www.pandemicflu.gov/ (online as of June 12, 2006).

Conclusions

This section summarizes our findings and conclusions in response to the three central research questions. It then discusses the implications of these conclusions for the future and provides recommendations.

How Has the Emerging Link Between Global Infectious Disease and U.S. National Security Been Perceived and Acted Upon Across Government Sectors?

Recent history of HIV/AIDS, SARS, and avian influenza H5N1, among other infectious diseases, has demonstrated once again the broad effects that "health" problems, specifically infectious diseases, can have on trade, economies, and social and political stability and, hence, on the national and global security of the United States and countries around the world. The threats posed by infectious disease have traditionally been considered strictly through a public health and medical lens. Similarly, the intelligence community has addressed a wide range of threats that heretofore has not fundamentally included health and infectious diseases. However, events evolving over the past ten years and accelerated by the terror attacks of 2001 and the imminent threat of a human influenza pandemic have highlighted the potential for infectious diseases to threaten U.S. national security. This heightened awareness is indicative of the link between the globalization of the world's economies and the spread of infectious diseases. As detailed in Chapter Three, these relationships have been confirmed by our review of the literature, and virtually all the stakeholders we interviewed clearly understood the new paradigm linking infectious disease to national security. With regard to collecting and using disease-related information, "business as usual" is no longer possible. The health sector is now obliged to address global infectious diseases from a broader context that includes national security, and the health sector will likely look increasingly to the intelligence community in order to collect needed and relevant information.

The U.S. government has begun to operationalize this new paradigm through security-oriented initiatives, such as those described in Chapters Two and Three and synthesized in the preceding section above. A now-broader community of stakeholders must find ways to combine their various expertise, methods, and perspectives to facilitate coherent and responsible action across government sectors to address the broad range of consequences associated with global infectious disease.

What Types of Information About Global Infectious Disease Do U.S. Policymakers Need?

Stakeholders from across a wide range of disciplines and sectors, including health, agriculture, foreign affairs, homeland security, and intelligence, have expressed the need for timely, accurate, complete, and understandable information that is delivered in a way that meets a wide range of requirements and does not overwhelm. These requirements range from technical disease and surveillance data to information about the social and political contexts related to outbreaks and subsequent responses. They range from raw data to synthesized analysis products, and from "push" to "pull" mechanisms of delivery.

While each sector has its own focus and responsibilities, the information needs of policymakers across sectors were characterized more by their similarities than by their differences.

The stakeholders we interviewed expressed a strong desire for a centralized system that provides needed information to all stakeholders. An ideal system to collect, analyze, and disseminate infectious disease information would be (1) robust, drawing information from a wide range of sources and collecting information that is accurate and complete; (2) efficient, constituting a single, integrated source of timely information available to all stakeholders; (3) tailored to meet individual stakeholder needs and preferences; and (4) accessible, notwithstanding the need for protection of sensitive data.

How Sufficient Is the Available Information on Global Infectious Diseases?

While there may never be enough good information to meet all legitimate policy needs, there is considerable information already available via open sources, complemented by protected information. Chapter Five describes the characteristics of the 234 online sources we compiled for this study. Our database alone can be useful to some policymakers, but it may never be sufficient, since online sources are added frequently and even 234 sources can be somewhat overwhelming. The organization and delivery of information thus poses a major challenge: It must be sufficiently complete while not overwhelming. The variety of information-gathering techniques, which now includes active Web crawling in addition to more standard disease reporting techniques, and the addition of intelligence collection methods, adds to the timeliness, breadth, and value of the overall body of information available to policymakers. There are new efforts to address information requirements centrally in order to serve needs more broadly across the federal government. One such effort is NBIS. Such efforts must focus on both data content and data coordination, i.e., they must be well integrated across agencies to support national goals. They must also be versatile enough to meet the wide range of policymakers' needs. The need for versatility suggests that a carefully managed system involving human analysts and experts is preferable to a solution based purely on information technology. Again, NBIS is intended to have such versatility. However, because NBIS is only in its early stages of implementation, it is too early to reach conclusions regarding the sufficiency of available information that NBIS may collect, process, and disseminate. There does not appear to be any other source that satisfies the full range of desired criteria expressed by the stakeholders we interviewed.

Implications and Remaining Challenges

Globalization of the world's economy has given rise to the globalization of infectious diseases and the need for a global approach to control them. Countries around the world require timely, accurate, and complete information on infectious diseases, presented in a way that is both understandable and actionable. Ideally, disease emergence and spread would be prevented altogether; if not, as is more likely, early warning indicators need to be followed and disease occurrences detected promptly so that appropriate actions can be taken to control their spread. Realizing this goal will require an understanding of diseases and information collection and analysis methods by a broad range of stakeholders.

Remaining challenges include not only efforts to collect more and better infectious disease information but also the efficient and effective integration and sharing of information across government sectors that have, at best, a relatively short history of working together on shared priorities. Thus, challenges include not only the type and amount of information that is needed but also the processes to share and make most effective use of such information across government sectors.

It was suggested by some stakeholders during this study that the United States needs a novel system for collecting, analyzing, and disseminating infectious disease information. Indeed, this need was an original hypothesis of this study. Like many of the stakeholders we interviewed, we were unaware of NBIS at the start of this study. Based on information we collected during the study, it seems that NBIS is intended to address many of the issues identified by policymakers. First, NBIS seeks to create an information technology platform to integrate data input from disparate sources, including extant U.S. information systems. Second, it seeks to integrate data analysis across sources and sectors, including anticipatory analyses. Third, it seeks to provide expert analysis of the integrated data by a team of interagency analysts. The extent to which NBIS fulfills these criteria and meets government-wide infectious disease information requirements and the expectations set by Congress will determine whether it ultimately provides sufficient information to policymakers.

Recommendations

Based on this study, our primary recommendation is for the implementation of a U.S. governmentwide system that provides timely, accurate, complete (i.e., integrated and sufficiently comprehensive), and understandable information on infectious disease threats and occurrences, presented and delivered in ways that are most convenient and usable to a wide range of policymakers. At this time, a recommendation of an entirely new infectious disease information system would be imprudent; a new system, NBIS, has already been funded but has not yet been fully implemented and evaluated. Rather, at this time, we recommend a systematic formative evaluation of NBIS to help ensure that NBIS is designed to fulfill all critical requirements and is implemented as designed. A subsequent summative evaluation can ascertain whether NBIS is adequate or whether new or different strategies are needed to collect, analyze, and deliver infectious disease information to the broad range of policymakers responsible for addressing infectious disease security threats to the United States. The following illustrative questions highlight issues we consider relevant to a near-term evaluation of NBIS. (The final question pertains to the proposed summative evaluation.)

- Are there remaining technological issues that need to be resolved to fully implement NBIS; i.e., is further research needed?
- How is NBIS integrated with other information and analysis systems?
- What authorities are required and exercised, and by whom, for collection-tasking?
- Is an appropriate leadership mechanism in place to coordinate efforts across sectors?
- Are other agencies
  - aware of NBIS authority?
  - appropriately resourced?
  - ready to integrate their own systems into NBIS?

- What are the long-term requirements for
  - interagency support and processes?
  - updating types of needed information and products?
- How can accessibility (classification) issues be resolved?
- Are there valuable lessons from other interagency initiatives, particularly in the area of effective cooperation and coordination across government sectors?
- Will NBIS meet the information needs articulated by stakeholders and described in this report?

Organizations Interviewed

This appendix lists the organizations with which our 53 stakeholder interviewees were affiliated. Our semistructured interview guide is presented in Appendix B.

U.S. Federal Organizations

Department of Agriculture
Animal and Plant Health Inspection Service
Foreign Agricultural Service

Department of Defense
Defense Threat Reduction Agency
Deputy Assistant Secretary of Defense for Chemical and Biological Defense
Office of the Assistant Secretary of Defense, Health Affairs
Uniformed Services University of the Health Sciences
U.S. Central Command
U.S. Pacific Command

Department of Health and Human Services
Centers for Disease Control and Prevention
Food and Drug Administration
Office of the Secretary
      Office of Global Health Affairs
      Office of Public Health Emergency Preparedness

Department of Homeland Security
Directorate of Science and Technology
National Biodefense Analysis and Countermeasures Center
National Biosurveillance Integration System

Department of State
Bureau of Arms Control
Bureau of Consular Affairs
Bureau of East Asian and Pacific Affairs/Bureau of Economic Policy/Asia-Pacific Economic
    Cooperation
Office of International Health Affairs
Office of the Medical Director

Intelligence Community
Central Intelligence Agency
National Intelligence Council

Peace Corps

White House
Homeland Security Council
Office of Science and Technology Policy

Other Organizations

Association of State and Territorial Health Officials
Georgia Department of Human Resources, Division of Public Health
Homeland Security Institute
RAND Corporation (former officials of the U.S. Departments of State, Defense, Health and
    Human Services, and the Agency for International Development)
World Health Organization

Interview Guide

We developed the following discussion guide for our semi-structured interviews. We used it as a general reference, selecting and tailoring the questions based on the organizational affiliation and level of each interviewee. We pilot tested the interviews with nine individuals (representatives of selected government offices, former federal officials now at RAND, and others), and then finalized the discussion guide based on these pilot interviews. Our results reflect the views of all persons interviewed, i.e., including those during the pilot phase. The research conducted during this study complied with RAND Human Subjects Committee policies and procedures.

1. In what ways, if any, are infectious diseases related to U.S. national security?
    1.1. What (kinds of) infectious diseases pose a threat to the United States?
    1.2. Are there specific characteristics of these diseases that make them a threat?
    1.3. What is the interest of your organization in addressing these disease threats, and why?
    1.4. Does your organization have a specific mandate to address these disease threats?

2. What kind of information related to global infectious diseases does your organization need?
    2.1. What information do you collect or receive?
    2.2. What gaps, if any, exist between information you need and what you already have or can collect?
    2.3. What is the primary purpose for collecting or receiving this information?
    2.4. How is the information analyzed?
    2.5. What product is produced from this information, and to whom is it presented?
    2.6. Has this product influenced policy decisions? If not, why? Would different/additional information or analysis have had a different influence?
    2.7. Address these same questions specifically for these cases: SARS, avian influenza, and the next as yet unknown emerging or reemerging disease.

3. Are there specific disease or infectious disease problems that worry you in terms of their emergence or reemergence?
    3.1. What actions are you taking to track these diseases or problems?
    3.2. How are you using the information you obtain?

4. What criteria would you consider most important for setting your organization's strategic infectious disease information needs? Please rate the following on a scale of zero to 10:
   - Geographic location/distribution of disease threat
   - (Low) likelihood of timely reporting by country of origin
   - Number of cases (i.e., few versus many)
   - Endemic (expected) versus epidemic (unexpected)
   - Source of pathogen/disease (air, food, water, zoonosis, etc.)
   - Possibility of malicious intent (bioterrorism)
   - Severity of disease/problem (morbidity, mortality)
   - (Poor) local public health/medical capacity to control spread
   - Potential for spread to other countries
   - Potential for spread to the United States
   - Ability to detect and control the disease in the United States
   - Availability and cost of effective treatment in the United States
   - Potential for disruption to foreign trade and economies
   - Potential for disruption to U.S. trade and economy
   - U.S. political concern
   - National security concern (if not captured above)
   - Other

5. Is sufficient information already available about global infectious diseases?
   5.1. What information sources does your organization currently use to collect or receive information on infectious diseases?
   5.2. Are you able to control the information coming into your organization?
   5.3. Are you able to task intelligence collection?

6. What kind of global infectious disease information is not publicly available, and under what circumstances?
   6.1. Is the current system of "honest reporting" of global infectious disease information sufficient for U.S. national security interests?

7. What delivery format and system for infectious disease information is most useful to your organization for strategic and tactical purposes?

8. Do you have specific suggestions regarding how to obtain additional needed information or make better use of existing information?

9. Do you believe that the United States should change the way it collects, analyzes, and considers information about global infectious diseases?
   9.1. How would you label such a system?
   9.2. If a change is warranted, please explain and describe the key features of recommended changes.

List of Online Sources

This appendix lists 234 online sources related to the detection, surveillance, and dissemination of information on infectious diseases and infectious disease outbreaks. The list is not intended to be exhaustive but serves to demonstrate the variety of open- and restricted-access sources available for these purposes. All data in the table are current as of the period in which data were collected for this study, July through October 2005.

Table C.1
List of Online Sources

	Name	Sponsor	Location	Brief Description	Access
			Multilateral Organizations—Global		
1	Food and Agriculture Organization of the United Nations (FAO) Livestock Disease Surveillance Manual	FAO	http://www.fao.org/DOCREP/004/X3331E/X3331E00.HTM	Manual on livestock disease surveillance and information systems	Open
2	Regional Animal Disease Surveillance and Control Network (RADISCON)	FAO	http://www.fao.org/ag/aga/agah/id/radiscon/Database.htm	A joint FAO/International Fund for Agricultural Development (IFAD) endeavor (since June 1996) targeting 29 nations located in North Africa, the Sahel, the Horn of Africa, the Middle East, and the Arab Gulf. RADISCON aims to promote animal disease surveillance within and among countries. Standardized data input includes RADISCON Disease Outbreak Report (RADDOR), RADISCON Monthly Report (RADM); integrated national, regional and international veterinary information system compatible and complementary to the FAO Emergency Prevention System (EMPRES) and the Office International des Epizoöties global systems	Open
3	Filariasis Surveillance	Global Alliance to Eliminate Lymphatic Filariasis	http://www.filariasis.org/index.pl?iid=2377	Provides data and supporting documents for the Program to Eliminate Lymphatic Filariasis (PELF)	Open
4	Office International des Epizoöties (OIE)	OIE	http://www.oie.int/eng/en_index.htm	Required international reporting of animal diseases; collects and disseminates the information gathered by national surveillance programs on epizootic diseases; includes alerts, weekly and monthly reports, inter alia	Open
5	OIE Animal Disease Data—Handistatus II Database	OIE	http://www.oie.int/hs2/report.asp?lang=en	Database organized chronologically and by country, containing information on "List A" and "List B" animal diseases that have serious consequences for international trade or public health	Open
6	OIE Standards on Antimicrobial Resistance	OIE	http://www.oie.int/eng/publicat/Ouvrages/a_119.htm	Ordering and abstract page for the OIE standards book for antimicrobial resistance research	Open

Table C.1—Continued

Name	Sponsor	Location	Brief Description	Access
7 Arab Ministries of Health Database	United Nations Educational, Scientific, and Cultural Organisation (UNESCO)	http://www.unesco.org/webworld/portal_bib/Libraries/Health/Arab_States/index.shtml	List of links to Arab ministries of health (or similar-level institutions)	Open
8 United Nations statistical database on refugees	United Nations High Commissioner for Refugees (UNHCR)	http://www.unhcr.ch/cgi-bin/texis/vtx/statistics	Data, trends, and statistical reports on refugees, asylum-seekers, returned refugees, and internally displaced and stateless persons in more than 150 countries	Open
9 World Health Organization (WHO) Global Influenza Surveillance/FluNet	WHO	http://www.who.int/entity/csr/disease/influenza/surveillance/en/index.html	Serves as a global alert mechanism for the emergence of influenza viruses with pandemic potential.	Registration
10 WHO drug resistance information	WHO	http://www.who.int/drug resistance/surveillance/en/	Gateway page for the WHO program to assist countries in instituting antimicrobial resistance surveillance	Open
11 WHO Disease Outbreak News	WHO	http://www.who.int/csr/don/en/	Posts alerts on confirmed worldwide disease outbreaks; input: diseases versus syndromes (mostly diseases)	Open
12 WHO outbreak verification list	WHO	http://www.who.int/csr/alertresponse/verification/en/index.html	Unofficial WHO distribution list to inform 800 selected subscribers about infectious disease outbreak threats	Authorization
13 WHO Global Outbreak Alert and Response Network (GOARN)	WHO	http://www.who.int/csr/outbreaknetwork/en/	A technical collaboration of existing institutions and networks that pool human and technical resources for the rapid identification, confirmation, and response to outbreaks of international importance	Authorization
14 WHO Weekly Epidemiological Report	WHO	http://www.who.int/wer/en/	Provides rapid and accurate dissemination of epidemiological information on cases and outbreaks of diseases	Open
15 WHO Antimicrobial Resistance Information Bank	WHO	http://oms2_b3e.jussieu.fr/arinfobank/	Interactive resource that is open to all to access and contribute to the global understanding of antimicrobial resistance as a public health problem	Open

Table C.1—Continued

Name	Sponsor	Location	Brief Description	Access
16 WHO disease outbreak archives by country	WHO	http://www.who.int/csr/don/archive/country/en/	Site cataloging of worldwide disease outbreaks by country	Open
17 WHO Disease outbreak archives by year	WHO	http://www.who.int/csr/don/archive/year/en/	Site cataloging worldwide disease outbreaks by year	Open
18 WHO Communicable Disease Surveillance and Response	WHO	http://www.who.int/csr/en/	Tracks and responds to the evolving infectious disease situation	Registration
19 WHO Global Atlas of Infectious Disease	WHO	http://globalatlas.who.int	In a single electronic platform, brings together for analysis and comparison standardized data and statistics for infectious diseases at country, regional, and global levels	Open
20 WHO Supranational Reference Laboratory Network for Drug-Resistant Tuberculosis	WHO	http://www.who.int/drugresistance/tb/labs/en/	National Reference Laboratories conducting quality-assured drug susceptibility testing in conjunction with national or area anti-TB drug resistance (antimicrobial resistance) surveillance	Open
21 WHO Global Network for Eradication of Polio/Measles	WHO; United Nations Children's Fund (UNICEF); U.S. Department of Health and Human Services (HHS)/Centers for Disease Control and Prevention (CDC)	http://www.polioeradication.org/	Describes the Global Polio Eradication Initiative (GPEI), spearheaded by national governments, the WHO, Rotary International, the CDC, and UNICEF	Open
22 Guinea Worm Surveillance	WHO, HHS/CDC, UNICEF	http://www.who.int/ctd/dracun/strategies.htm	General information on Guinea Worm–related disease, surveillance information, and network	Open
23 Global Environment Monitoring System/Food Contamination Monitoring and Assessment Programme (GEMS/Food)	WHO	http://www.who.int/foodsafety/chem/gems/en/index5.html	Compiles food contamination monitoring data in Europe	Open

Table C.1—Continued

Name	Sponsor	Location	Brief Description	Access
24 Global Salm-Surv (GSS)	WHO; Danish Institute for Food and Veterinary Research (DFVF); HHS/CDC; Institut Pasteur; Public Health Agency, Canada; Animal Sciences Health Group, Wageningen University and Research Centre	http://www.who.int/salmsurv/en/	Facilitates communication and data exchange between labs that isolate, identify, and test specimens for salmonella in order to improve the quality and capacity of testing	Open
Multilateral Organizations—Regional				
25 Southeast Asian Nations Infectious Diseases Outbreak Surveillance Network	Association of Southeast Asian Nations (ASEAN) Secretariat; Ministry of Health, Republic of Indonesia	http://www.asean-disease-surveillance.net/ASNSurveillance.asp?Country=sg	Infectious Disease Surveillance network for ASEAN and three member organizations	Registration
26 Emerging Infections Network (EINet)	Asia-Pacific Economic Cooperation (APEC)	http://depts.washington.edu/einet/?a=home	A forum for reporting, discussion, and dissemination of information regarding unusual infectious disease cases/outbreaks in the Asia-Pacific region, and emerging infectious disease–related papers and meetings	Open
27 Enter-Net, formerly known as Salm-Net	European Commission	http://www.hpa.org.uk/hpa/inter/enter-net_menu.htm	International surveillance network for human gastrointestinal infections	Open
28 EuroTB	European Commission	http://www.eurotb.org/	Coordinates the surveillance of TB and TB antimicrobial resistance in the 52 countries of the WHO European region since 1996; its overall aim is to improve the contribution of epidemiological surveillance to TB control in Europe.	Authorization
29 Directory of European Disease Surveillance Systems	European Commission, Public Health Section	http://europa.eu.int/comm/health/ph_threats/com/comm_diseases_networks_en.htm	Directory of links to surveillance systems in the European region for communicable diseases	Open

Table C.1—Continued

Name	Sponsor	Location	Brief Description	Access
30	European Influenza Surveillance Scheme (EISS)	European Commission	http://www.eiss.org/	EISS collects and exchanges timely information on influenza activity in Europe; most clinical influenza surveillance is based on reports from sentinel general practitioners and sentinel pediatricians and physicians with other specializations. (Sentinel physicians usually represent 1–5% of physicians working in the country or region.) During the influenza season, clinical and virological data are collected on a weekly basis by each participating network. The data are processed, analyzed, and assessed before being entered into the EISS online database, available for query and analysis to authorized members.	Authorization
31	Eurosurveillance	European Centre for Disease Prevention and Control (ECDC)	http://www.eurosurveillance.org/releases/index-02.asp	Peer-reviewed information on communicable disease surveillance and control across Europe	Open
32	European Union public health Web site	European Union	http://europa.eu.int/pol/health/index_en.htm	Gateway site to European Union activities related to public health	Open
33	WHO, Regional Office for Africa (WHO-AFRO)	WHO/AFRO	http://www.afro.who.int/csr	Provides reporting on Africa-centric health issues, bulletins, and other programmatic content	Open
34	Integrated Disease Surveillance (IDS) and Epidemic Preparedness and Response Project	WHO/AFRO	http://www.afro.who.int/csr/ids/	Contributes to the improvement of epidemic preparedness and response and to the control of communicable diseases in the Africa region	Open
35	WHO, Regional Office for Europe, Centralized Information System for Infectious Diseases (CSID)	WHO/EURO	http://data.euro.who.int/cisid	Centralized information system for infectious diseases; uses advanced technology to collect, analyze, and present data on infectious diseases in the WHO European region	Authorization
36	WHO Surveillance Program for the Control of Foodborne Infections and Intoxicants in Europe	WHO/EURO	http://www.euro.who.int/eprise/main/WHO/Progs/FOS/Surveillance/20020903_3	Monitors and registers foodborne diseases and contamination	Open

Table C.1—Continued

Name	Sponsor	Location	Brief Description	Access
37 Caribbean Epidemiology Center (CAREC) disease surveillance system	WHO/Pan American Health Organization (PAHO)	http://www.carec.org/ publications/reg-pub. html#surveil	Research, training, and advocacy organization based in Trinidad and Tobago that concentrates on statistical and laboratory research, analysis, and reporting, as well as training for citizens of regional members in the practicum of public health	Open
38 PAHO Antimicrobial Resistance	WHO/PAHO	http://www.paho.org/english/ hcp/hct/eer/antimicrob.htm	PAHO homepage for antimicrobial resistance; includes surveillance, prevention and control, activities, and materials	Open
39 Eurosurveillance European national bulletins	ECDC	http://www.eurosurveillance. org/links/links-05.asp# bulletinsEU	Directory of links to surveillance summaries for communicable diseases in the European region	Open
National—U.S.				
40 California Electronic Laboratory Disease Alert and Reporting (CELDAR) system	California Department of Health Services (DHS)	URL not available	Laboratory-based surveillance of reportable diseases in California	Authorization
41 California Influenza Surveillance Project (CISP)	California DHS, Division of Communicable Disease Control; HHS/CDC; Kaiser Permanente	http://www.dhs.ca.gov/ps/ dcdc/VRDL/html/FLU/Fluintro. htm	Reflects statewide influenza surveillance year-round; weekly updates of the Web site occur during influenza season	Open
42 Foreign Broadcast Information Service (FBIS) (now Open Source Center)	Central Intelligence Agency (CIA)	https://www.fbis.gov/	Provides translated foreign media reporting and analysis to policymakers, government institutions, and strategic partners	Authorization
43 U.S. Census Bureau International Data Base	U.S. Census Bureau	http://www.census.gov/ipc/ www/idbnew.html	Statistical tables of demographic and socioeconomic data for 227 countries and areas of the world	Open
44 Data Web	U.S. Census Bureau; HHS/CDC	http://www.thedataweb.org/	Network of data libraries focused on demographic, economic, environmental, health, and other data already collected by a variety of U.S. organizations	Open

Table C.1—Continued

Name	Sponsor	Location	Brief Description	Access
45 Lower Echelon Reporting and Surveillance Module (LERSM)	U.S. Department of Defense (DoD)	http://www.tricare.osd.mil/peo/tmip/programs.htm	LERSM provides a query capability to the local medical treatment facility (MTF) commander based on information collected at that location; when this information is analyzed, the local MTF commander will be able to take preventive actions to further protect individual soldiers	Authorization
46 Defense Medical Logistics Standard Support (DMLSS)	Office of the Secretary of Defense (Health Affairs); Joint Medical Logistics Functional Development Center	http://www.tricare.osd.mil/dmlss/more_info.cfm	Provides automation support of reengineered medical logistics business practices and delivers a comprehensive range of materiel, equipment, and facilities management information systems; DMLSS is an Acquisition Category 1A acquisition program	Authorization
47 Disease Occurrence Worldwide (DOW)	DoD/Armed Forces Medical Intelligence Center (AFMIC)	http://mic.afmic.detrick.army.mil/	DOW is a monthly summary of disease occurrences of military importance.	Authorization
48 DOD-GEIS (Global Emergency Infections System), Asia-Pacific Disease Outbreak/Surveillance Reports	DoD-GEIS	http://www.geis.fhp.osd.mil/GEIS/SurveillanceActivities/apdosr/apdosrmenu.asp	Asia-Pacific Disease Outbreak/Surveillance Reports	Open
49 DoD-GEIS Antimicrobial Resistance	DoD-GEIS	http://www.geis.fhp.osd.mil/GEIS/SurveillanceActivities/AntiMicrobialResistance/AR-surveillance.asp	Program for the development of a DoD-wide surveillance mechanism for identifying antimicrobial resistance occurrences and trends within the U.S. military force using The Surveillance Network® (TSN®); U.S. military locations	Open
50 DoD Influenza Surveillance Program (formerly known as Project Gargle)	DoD-GEIS	http://www.geis.fhp.osd.mil/GEIS/SurveillanceActivities/Influenza/influenza.asp	Goals are to detect local respiratory outbreaks, provide isolates to the WHO, and detect emerging strains	Authorization
51 Military Public Health Laboratories	DoD-GEIS; Armed Forces Institute of Pathology (APHIP)	http://www.geis.fhp.osd.mil/GEIS/SurveillanceActivities/AFIP/directory.asp	Provides information on these laboratories as part of the development of regional surveillance networks	Authorization
52 Theater Medical Information Program (TMIP)	Office of the Secretary of Defense (Health Affairs)	http://www.tricare.osd.mil/peo/tmip/default.htm	Integrates DoD's "peacetime" medical software and tailors it to run on a combination of handheld devices, stand-alone laptop	Authorization

Table C.1—Continued

	Name	Sponsor	Location	Brief Description	Access
53	Joint Biological Agent Identification and Diagnostic System (JBAIDS)	DoD/Joint Program Executive Office for Chemical and Biological Defense	http://www.jpeocbd.osd.mil/MS_JBAIDS.htm	An integrated system for the rapid identification and diagnostic confirmation of biological agent exposure or infection	Authorization
54	Electronic Surveillance System for the Early Notification of Community-based Epidemics (ESSENCE)	DoD/U.S. Army	URL not available	ESSENCE provides population-based monitoring and an early warning capability of a potential chemical or biological attack on or near a military installation.	Authorization
55	Army Medical Surveillance Activity (AMSA)	DoD/U.S. Army, Center for Health Promotion and Preventive Medicine (USACHPPM)	http://amsa.army.mil/AMSA/amsa_home.htm	Performs comprehensive medical surveillance and routinely publishes background rates of diseases and injuries for the Army population	Authorization
56	Early Warning Outbreak Recognition System (EWORS)	DoD/U.S. Navy	http://www.apha.confex.com/	A hospital-based network of computerized linkages that provides surveillance for early detection of infectious disease outbreaks by establishing trend information that distinguishes epidemic from endemic diseases	Authorization
57	Medical Surveillance Monthly Report (MSMR)	DoD/USACHPPM	http://amsa.army.mil/AMSA/AMSA_MSMROverview.htm	The U.S. Army Medical Surveillance Activity's (AMSA) principal vehicle for disseminating medical surveillance information of broad interest	Open
58	Defense Occupational and Environmental Health Readiness System (DOEHRS)	DoD/USACHPPM	http://chppm-www.apgea.army.mil/IndustrialHygiene/DOEHRS.aspx	Records contain a history of individual worker pre-deployment, deployment, and post-deployment exposures; the data can then be analyzed and utilized by practitioners to prioritize preventive medicine actions	Authorization
59	Medical Situational Awareness–Advanced Concept Technology Demonstrator (MSAT-ACTD)	DoD/U.S. Army Medical Research and Materiel Command (USAMRMC)	https://fhp.osd.mil/msat/index.jsp	Uses current and emerging technologies and applies artificial intelligence and computerized decision-support systems to transform collected, scattered data into timely, actionable information for combatant commanders	Authorization

Table C.1—Continued

Name	Sponsor	Location	Brief Description	Access
60	Battlefield Medical Information System (BMIST)	DoD/USAMRMC, Telemedicine and Advanced Technology (TATRC), U.S. Special Operations Command (USSOCOM)	https://www.mc4.army.mil/HTML/BMIST-J.asp	An application used on a point-of-care handheld assistant, enabling medics and front-line providers to record, store, retrieve, and transmit the essential elements of patient encounters in an operational setting	Authorization
61	Joint Medical Workstation (JMeWS)	DoD/U.S. Central Command (USCENTCOM), Defense Information Systems Agency (DISA)	http://acq.osd.mil/actd/articles/JMEWS.doc	Enables commanders and medical personnel to note trends and collect data on the health of service members, and provides information on medical treatment facilities, such as stock of blood available	Authorization
62	Epidemic Outbreak Surveillance (EOS) system	DoD/U.S. Joint Forces Command (USJFCOM), U.S. Air Force Surgeon General (USAF/SG)	http://www.jfcom.mil/newslink/storyarchive/2004/pa040504.htm	A proposed advanced concept technology demonstrator (ACTD) sponsored by the USJFCOM command surgeon with the USAF/SG; detects viruses days earlier than conventional methods	Authorization
63	Shipboard Non-Tactical Automated Medical System (SAMS)	DoD/U.S. Navy	http://www.mhs-helpdesk.com/Pages/SAMS.asp	A versatile, automated medical support application developed to improve naval health care by reducing the administrative burden on health care providers (ship-based)	Authorization
64	Medical Data Surveillance System (MDSS)	DoD/U.S. Navy, U.S. Marine Corps (USMC)	http://www.stormingmedia.us/57/5753/A575334.html	Designed and developed as a Web-enabled system for data analysis and reporting for the medical surveillance of Navy and Marine Corps deployed forces; the primary objective of the system is to rapidly detect medical threats from the analysis of routine patient data	Authorization
65	LandScan	U.S. Department of Energy (DOE)/ Oakridge National Laboratory	http://www.ornl.gov/sci/gist/landscan/	Provides detailed worldwide population information for estimating ambient populations at risk during hazardous releases (e.g., chemical, biological, radiological)	Subscription
66	Bio-Detection Systems	HHS/Agency for Healthcare Research and Quality (AHRQ)	http://www.ahrq.gov/downloads/pub/evidence/pdf/bioit/evtbls.pdf	List of biodetection systems for four categories of detection systems: collection systems, particulate counters and biomass indicators, identification systems, and integrated collection and identification systems	Open

Table C.1—Continued

	Name	Sponsor	Location	Brief Description	Access
67	Rapid Syndrome Validation Project (RSVP)	DOE/Sandia and Los Alamos National Laboratories; University of New Mexico; New Mexico Office of Epidemiology	http://www.ca.sandia.gov/chembio/implementation_proj/rsvp/	Provides medical (syndromic) surveillance and rapid communication by clinicians in a variety of clinical areas	Authorization
68	National Guideline Clearinghouse™ (NGC)	HHS/AHRQ; American Medical Association; American Association of Health Plans	http://www.guideline.gov/	A public resource for evidence-based clinical practice guidelines; it is a clearinghouse of clinical practice guidelines on wide-ranging topics in clinical medicine	Open
69	CDC Gonococcal Isolate Surveillance Project	HHS/CDC	http://www.cdc.gov/ncidod/dastlr/gcdir/Resist/gisp.html	Monitors antimicrobial resistance in Neisseria gonorrhoeae in the United States	Open
70	Global Laboratory Network for Measles Surveillance	HHS/CDC	http://www.cdc.gov/ncidod/dvrd/revb/measles/index.htm	Facilitates communication among laboratories that conduct measles diagnosis and virus characterization, as well as those involved in the surveillance of measles	Open
71	National Malaria Surveillance System	HHS/CDC	http://www.cdc.gov/malaria/cdcactivities/nmss.htm	Collects epidemiological and clinical information on malaria cases diagnosed in the United States (vector) (notifiable disease)	Open
72	National Tuberculosis Genotyping and Surveillance Network	HHS/CDC	http://www.cdc.gov/ncidod/dastlr/TB/TB_TGSN.htm	Studies epidemiology of tuberculosis outbreaks via laboratory strain-typing	Open
73	CDC Bacterial Contamination of Blood Study	HHS/CDC	http://www.cdc.gov/ncidod/hip/bacon/index.htm	Study of adverse transfusion reactions suspected to be due to bacterial contamination of blood or blood products	Open
74	CDC Active Bacterial Core Surveillance	HHS/CDC	http://www.cdc.gov/ncidod/dbmd/abcs/default.htm	An active laboratory- and population-based surveillance system for invasive bacterial pathogens of public health importance	Open
75	Public Health Information Network (PHIN)	HHS/CDC	http://www.cdc.gov/phin/index.html	A national initiative to implement a multi-organizational business and technical architecture for public health information systems	Authorization

Table C.1—Continued

Name	Sponsor	Location	Brief Description	Access
76 Unexplained Deaths and Critical Illnesses Surveillance System	HHS/CDC	http://www.cdc.gov/ncidod/eid/vol8no2/01-0165.htm	Improves the CDC's capacity to rapidly identify the causes of unexplained deaths or critical illnesses and to improve understanding of the causes of specific infectious disease syndromes for which an etiologic agent is frequently not identified	Open
77 Environmental Public Health Tracking (EPHT) Network	HHS/CDC	http://www.cdc.gov/nceh/tracking/network.htm	Ongoing collection, integration, analysis, interpretation, and dissemination of data from environmental hazard monitoring and from human exposure and health-effects surveillance	Authorization
78 Health Alert Network (HAN)	HHS/CDC	http://www.phppo.cdc.gov/han/	A secure Web-based information and communication system designed by the CDC to link local and state public health agencies with each other and with other organizations responsible for responding to a bioterrorism attack	Authorization
79 Epidemic Information Exchange (Epi-X)	HHS/CDC	http://www.cdc.gov/mmwr/epix.html	Provides secure Web-based communication and information functions for use in both routine and emergency public health situations	Authorization
80 International Network for the Study and Prevention of Emerging Antimicrobial Resistance (INSPEAR)	HHS/CDC	http://www.cdc.gov/ncidod/hip/surveill/inspear.HTM	Main purposes in the hospital/health care facility are to (1) serve as an early warning system for emerging antimicrobial resistance, (2) rapidly distribute information about this resistance, and (3) serve as a model for the development and implementation of infection-control interventions	Authorization
81 National Electronic Telecommunications System for Surveillance (NETSS)	HHS/CDC	http://www.cdc.gov/epo/dphsi/netss.htm	System for reporting notifiable disease and injury reports from participating health agencies (and U.S. territories) to state health departments and the CDC	Authorization
82 CDC Morbidity and Mortality Weekly Report (MMWR)	HHS/CDC	http://www.cdc.gov/mmwr	Comprehensive source of information-reporting at different time intervals and on diverse disease-related issues in the United States and abroad	Open
83 Electronic Foodborne Outbreak Reporting System (EFORS)	HHS/CDC	http://www.cdc.gov/foodborneoutbreaks/index.htm	Investigates outbreaks and establishes both short-term control measures and long-term improvements to prevent similar outbreaks in the future	Open

Table C.1—Continued

Name		Sponsor	Location	Brief Description	Access
84	National West Nile Virus Surveillance System (ArboNET)	HHS/CDC	http://www.cdc.gov/ncidod/dvbid/westnile/surv&control.htm	Monitors the geographic and temporal spread of West Nile virus in humans and animals in the United States (i.e., birds and mosquitoes) (West Nile virus is not nationally notifiable)	Open
85	121 cities' mortality reporting system (122 cities participating)	HHS/CDC	http://www.cdc.gov/epo/dphsi/121hist.htm	Weekly mortality reports from 122 cities in the United States within 2–3 weeks from the date of death; total number of deaths occurring in these cities/areas each week, and number due to pneumonia and influenza	Open
86	National Nosocomial Infections Surveillance (NNIS) System	H-IS/CDC	http://www.cdc.gov/ncidod/hip/SURVEILL/NNIS.HTM	Collects nosocomial infection surveillance data that can be aggregated into a national database for monitoring of trends in infections and risk factors	Authorization
87	National Respiratory and Enteric Virus Surveillance System (NREVSS)	HHS/CDC	http://www.cdc.gov/ncidod/dvrd/revb/nrevss/	Monitors temporal and geographic patterns associated with the detection of respiratory and enteric viruses	Open
88	National Healthcare Survey (NHCS)	HHS/CDC	http://www.cdc.gov/nchs/nhcs.htm	Encompasses a family of health care provider surveys, obtaining information about the facilities that supply health care, the services rendered, and the characteristics of the patients served	Open
89	National Molecular Subtyping Network for Foodborne Disease Surveillance (PulseNet)	HHS/CDC	http://www.cdc.gov/ncidod/eid/vol7no3/swaminathan.htm	Creates a national molecular subtyping network for foodborne bacterial disease surveillance	Authorization
90	CDC Surveillance Systems Monitoring Infectious Diseases	HHS/CDC	http://www.cdc.gov/ncidod/osr/site/sentinel/surv-sys.htm	Page of links to disease surveillance programs nationwide	Open
91	United States Influenza Sentinel Physicians Surveillance Network	H-S/CDC	http://www.cdc.gov/flu/weekly/	Weekly report of U.S. influenza cases	Open
92	Dialysis Surveillance Network (DSN)	HHS/CDC	http://www.cdc.gov/ncidod/hip/DIALYSIS/dsn.htm	Monitors bloodstream and vascular infections at dialysis centers nationwide	Open

Table C.1—Continued

Name	Sponsor	Location	Brief Description	Access
93 National Surveillance System for Healthcare Workers (NaSH)	HHS/CDC	http://www.cdc.gov/ncidod/hip/SURVEILL/nash.htm	Allows the CDC to monitor trends, detect emerging occupational hazards, and evaluate prevention policies for infectious disease exposure of health care workers	Authorization
94 Laboratory Information Tracking System (LITS)	HHS/CDC	http://www.cdc.gov/ncidod/dbmd/litsplus/default.htm	Data management and laboratory specimen-tracking system; this page describes the system	Authorization
95 Waterborne-Disease Outbreak Surveillance System	HHS/CDC	http://www.cdc.gov/ncidod/osr/site/sentinel/surv-sys.htm	Collaborative surveillance system of the occurrences and causes of waterborne disease outbreaks.	Open
96 Laboratory Response Network	HHS/CDC	http://www.bt.cdc.gov/lrn/	Standardized nationwide public health laboratory network to improve response capabilities for a bioterrorism attack	Open
97 Foodborne Diseases Active Surveillance Network (FoodNet)	HHS/CDC, Food and Drug Administration (FDA); U.S. Department of Agriculture (USDA)	http://www.cdc.gov/foodnet/	Monitors foodborne diseases	Open
98 National Antimicrobial Resistance Monitoring System (NARMS)	HHS/CDC, FDA; USDA/Food Safety and Inspection Service (FSIS), Agricultural Research Service (ARS)	http://www.cdc.gov/narms/	Monitors antimicrobial resistance in human enteric pathogens	Open
99 National Prion Disease Surveillance	HHS/CDC, National Institutes of Health (NIH); American Association of Neuropathologists	http://www.cjdsurveillance.com (Case Western Reserve University)	Established as a surveillance center to monitor the occurrence of prion diseases, or spongiform encephalopathies, in response to the epidemic of bovine spongiform encephalopathy (BSE)	Open
100 Salmonella Outbreak Detection Algorithm (SODA)	HHS/CDC, National Center for Infectious Diseases (NCID)	http://www.cdc.gov/ncidod/dbmd/phlisdata/default.htm	Tracks, via serotyping and a statistical algorithm, outbreaks and clinical isolates of salmonella	Open
101 EMERGEncy ID NET	HHS/CD, National Center for Infectious Diseases	http://www.cdc.gov/Ncidod/osr/site/surv_resources/surv_sys.htm	An interdisciplinary, multicenter, emergency department–based network for research on emerging infectious diseases	Authorization

Table C.1—Continued

Name	Sponsor	Location	Brief Description	Access
102 Global Emerging Infections Sentinel Network (GeoSentinel)	HHS/CDC; International Society of Travel Medicine (ISTM)	http://www.istm.org/ geosentinel/main.html	A worldwide communication and data collection network for the surveillance of travel-related morbidity	Authorization
103 Lightweight Epidemiology Advanced Detection and Emergency Response System (LEADERS)	HHS/CDC; Oracle, Idaho Technology Inc.; Defense Advanced Research Projects Agency (DARPA)	http://www.scenpro.com/sec_ prod_leaders.html	Integrates a data collection, analysis, and management system for syndromal and other event-based surveillance for early detection of a bioterrorism event; can also track casualties, bed occupancy, and emergency department diversion status	Authorization
104 Surveillance for Emerging Antimicrobial Resistance Connected to Healthcare (SEARCH)	HHS/CDC, Division of Healthcare Quality Promotion (DHQP)	http://www.cdc.gov/ncidod/ dhqp/dprc_search.html	Monitors vancomycin-resistant S. aureus and provide confirmatory MIC testing when local testing is not feasible (antimicrobial resistance)	Authorization
105 National Electronic Disease Surveillance System (NEDSS)	HHS/CDC, PHIN	http://www.cdc.gov/nedss/	The surveillance/monitoring component of the Public Health Information Network; detects outbreaks rapidly and facilitates electronic data transfer from clinical information systems to public health departments	Authorization
106 BioSense Early Event Detection System	HHS/CDC, PHIN	http://www.cdc.gov/phin/ component-initiatives/ biosense/index.html	An initiative to improve U.S. capabilities for near–real-time disease detection by using data (without patient names or medical numbers) from existing health-related databases	Authorization
107 Composite Health Care System II—Theater (CHCS II-T)	DoD	http://www.mhs-helpdesk. com/Pages/chcsii-t.asp	Modified from CHCS II to provide clinical encounter functionality on a stand-alone laptop computer in a deployed theater environment	Authorization
108 Indianapolis Network for Patient Care (INPC)	HHS/NIH National Library of Medicine (through Regenstrief Institute for Healthcare)	http://www.inpc.org/ and five participating Indianapolis hospitals	The INPC is being created as a shared database storing emergency room encounter records, hospital abstracts, clinical laboratory data, and other data as available for use by emergency departments.	Authorization
109 HEALTHCOM	New York State Department of Health	http://www.health.state.ny.us/	Web-based communication system connecting county health departments of New York state	Authorization

Table C.1—Continued

Name	Sponsor	Location	Brief Description	Access
110 New York State Department of Health, Bureau of Community Sanitation and Food Protection (BCSFP)	New York State Department of Health	http://www.health.state.ny.us/	Homepage for NY Department of Health; multiple topics, including disease statistics, emergency preparedness and response, food preparation practices, etc.	Open
111 Syndromal Surveillance Tally Sheet	Santa Clara County, California, Department of Public Health	http://www.scvmed.org/scc/ assets/docs/92939Keyboard Transmittal-0048376.PDF	Reflects data from Santa Clara County, California	Authorization
112 Texas Department of State Health Services Infectious Disease Control Unit	Texas Department of State Health Services	http://www.tdh.state.tx.us/ ideas/about/overview/	Program assists local or regional public health officials in investigating and reporting outbreaks of acute infectious or rare diseases; conducts routine and special morbidity surveillance of diseases (Epi/ Surveillance homepage)	Open
113 USACHPPM Health Information Operations Weekly Update	DoD/USACHPPM	http://chppm-www.apgea. army.mil/Hioupdate/	Weekly news update on preventive medicine, environmental and occupational health, health promotion and wellness, epidemiology and disease surveillance, toxicology, and related laboratory sciences related to global medical and veterinary issues of interest	Open
114 U.S. Geological Survey Disease Surveillance Mapping	U.S. Geological Survey	http://wildlifedisease.nbii.gov/ Mapping/maps.html	Shows the available disease data in wild animal populations overlaid on a map of the United States	Open
115 USDA Foreign Agricultural Service (FAS)	USDA	http://www.fas.usda.gov/icd/ protecting.asp	Intended to help improve foreign market access for U.S. products and protecting the food supply	Open
116 Cornell University Pathogen Tracker 2.0	USDA; American Meat Institute Foundation	http://cbsusrv01.tc.cornell.edu/ users/PathogenTracker/pt2/ login/login.aspx	This internet database currently allows access to genetic, phenotypic, and source information of a collection of foodborne and zoonotic pathogens and food-spoilage organisms.	Authorization
117 National Bovine Spongiform Encephalopathy Testing Program	USDA/Animal and Plant Inspection Service (APHIS)	http://www.aphis.usda.gov/ lpa/issues/bse_testing/test_ results.html	Involves the use of a rapid screening test, followed by confirmatory testing for any samples that come back "inconclusive"	Open

Table C.1—Continued

	Name	Sponsor	Location	Brief Description	Access
118	Center for Emerging Issues (CEI) Impact Worksheets	USDA/APHIS	http://www.aphis.usda.gov/vs/ceah/cei/worksheets.htm	Assessment of disease occurrences in the United States and in foreign countries and threats to U.S. livestock	Open
119	APHIS Hot Issues Archive	USDA/APHIS	http://www.aphis.usda.gov/lpa/issues/issues.html	Issues considered to be of immediate interest by the USDA-APHIS, such as disease outbreaks and new discoveries	Open
120	National Animal Health Monitoring System (NAHMS)	USDA/APHIS	http://www.aphis.usda.gov/vs/ceah/ncahs/nahms/index.htm	Collects data on animal disease incidence and prevalence, mortality, management practices, and disease costs	Open
121	Vesicular Stomatitis Virus Surveillance	USDA/APHIS	http://www.aphis.usda.gov/vs/ceah/ncahs/nsu/surveillance/vsv/vsv.htm	Surveillance reports on vesicular stomatitis in U.S. states	Open
122	Food and Animal Residue Avoidance Databank (FARAD)	USDA/FSIS	http://www.farad.org/	A computerized databank of data necessary to solve a drug or chemical residue problem in food-producing animals	Open
123	Emerging Pathogens Initiative (EPI)	Department of Veterans Affairs (VA) Program for Infectious Diseases	http://www.nibs.org/FMOCVA.pdf	For surveillance of emerging pathogens in 172 VA health care facilities worldwide; pathogens: vancomycin-resistant enterococcus, penicillin-resistant pneumococcus, E. coli, candida bloodstream infections, Clostridium difficile, cryptosporidium, dengue, antibody-positive hepatitis C, legionella, leishmaniasis, malaria, and others.	Authorization
124	USAID Infectious Disease Programming	United States Agency for International Development (USAID)	http://www.usaid.gov/our_work/global_health/id/	Description and links to various USAID infectious disease programs and reports, including specific topics: malaria, TB, surveillance, antimicrobial resistance	Open
National—Foreign					
125	Hong Kong Government Disease Surveillance	Government of the People's Republic of China, Hong Kong Special Administrative Region	http://www.info.gov.hk/dh/diseases	For communicable diseases, the surveillance and epidemiology branch conducts surveillance on 30 statutorily notifiable diseases and other infections of public health significance.	Open

Table C.1—Continued

Name	Sponsor	Location	Brief Description	Access
126 Australia National Serology Reference Laboratory (NRL)	Govternment of Australia	http://www.nrl.gov.au/	Maintains quality in serological testing, particularly for retroviral and other bloodborne diseases and sets standards to provide accurate and cost-effective serological testing in screening	Open
127 Australian National Animal Health Information System (NAHIS)	Government of Australia/Animal Health	http://www. animalhealthaustralia.com. au/status/nahis.cfm	Monitors animals' health status and aids in decisionmaking	Open
128 Transmissible Spongiform Encephalopathy (TSE) Freedom Assurance Program Australia	Government of Australia/Animal Health	http://www. animalhealthaustralia.com. au/programs/adsp/tsefap/ tsefap_home.cfm	TSE Freedom Assurance Program homepage with TSE surveillance information	Open
129 Salmonella Potential Outbreak Targeting System (SPOT)/National Enteric Pathogens Surveillance Scheme (NEPSS)	Government of Australia/Department of Health and Ageing	http://www.health.gov.au/ internet/wcms/publishing.nsf/ Content/cda-surveil-surv_sys. htm#nepss	For early detection of potential salmonella outbreaks	Open
130 Australia Zoonotic Disease	Government of Australia/Departments of Health and Ageing and Agriculture, Fisheries, and Forestry	http://www.health.gov.au/ internet/wcms/publishing. nsf/Content/health- pubhlth-strateg-jetacar-pdf- amrstrategy_affa.htm	Pilot surveillance program for antimicrobial resistance in bacteria of animal origin; summary information and links to details	Open
131 Communicable Diseases Intelligence	Government of Australia/Department of Health and Ageing (Surveillance Section), Communicable Diseases and Biosecurity Branch	http://www.health.gov.au/ internet/wcms/Publishing. nsf/Content/cda-pubs-cdipubs. htm	Current surveillance intelligence on communicable diseases in Australia accompanied by interpretation and expert commentary	Open
132 Ministry of Health, Bahrain	Government of Bahrain	http://www.moh.gov.bh/	Ministry of health Web site containing information for the general public and preparedness information for health professionals	Open

Table C.1—Continued

Name	Sponsor	Location	Brief Description	Access
133 Ministry of Health, Botswana	Government of Botswana	http://www.moh.gov.bw/	Ministry of health Web site containing information for the general public and preparedness information for health professionals	Open
134 Animal Disease Surveillance Unit	Government of Canada/Food Inspection Agency	http://www.inspection.gc.ca/english/anima/surv/surve.shtml	A nationwide network known as CAHNet (Canadian Animal Health Network) unites the disease-detection capabilities of practicing veterinarians, provincial and university diagnostic laboratories, and the federal government.	Open
135 Global Public Health Intelligence Network (GPHIN)	Government of Canada/Health Canada; WHO	http://www.phac-aspc.gc.ca/	GPHIN's powerful search engines actively crawl the World Wide Web for reports on communicable diseases and syndromes.	Subscription
136 Canadian Disease Surveillance Directory	Government of Canada/Health Canada	http://www.hc-sc.gc.ca/dc-ma/surveill/index_e.html	Enhances infection-prevention and -control programs in health care facilities and other community settings by collecting, analyzing, interpreting, and disseminating information related to diseases and conditions	Open
137 Canada Communicable Disease Report (CCDR)	Government of Canada/Health Canada	http://www.phac-aspc.gc.ca/publicat/ccdr-rmtc/05vol31/index.html	Presents current information on infectious and other diseases for surveillance purposes	Subscription
138 Notifiable Diseases On-Line	Government of Canada/PHAC	http://dsol-smed.phac-aspc.gc.ca/dsol-smed/ndis/c_ind_e.html#top_list	Database for cases of notifiable diseases in Canada by province, age, and sex	Open
139 Canadian Integrated Program for Antimicrobial Resistance Surveillance (CIPARS)	Government of Canada/Public Health Agency of Canada (PHAC)	http://www.phac-aspc.gc.ca/cipars-picra/	Information is being collected on resistance in enteric pathogens and commensal organisms from the agri-food sector, in enteric pathogens isolated from humans, and on antimicrobial use in humans and animals.	Open
140 Danish National Hospital Discharge Registry	Government of Denmark/National Board of Health	http://www.sst.dk/Informatik_og_sundhedsdata/Registre_og_sundhedsstatistik/Beskrivelse_af_registre/Landspatientregister.aspx?lang=en	Develops a discharge registry of all patients admitted to Danish hospitals (except psychiatric); an algorithm was developed to see if data source is useful for surveillance	Authorization

Table C.1—Continued

Name	Sponsor	Location	Brief Description	Access
141 Institute de Veille Sanitaire (INVS)	Government of France	http://www.invs.sante.fr/beh	INVS, a public establishment, under the Ministry for Health and the Family, has the role of supervising the health of the whole of the population, and of alerting the authorities in the event of threat to the public health in France	Open
142 SentiWeb	Government of France/Department of Health, National Institute of Health and Medical Research (INSERM)	http://rhone.b3e.jussieu.fr/senti/	Web-based reporting of weekly sentinel reports on communicable diseases in France	Open
143 Arbeitsgemeinschaft Influenza (AGI) Sentinel Surveillance System	Government of Germany; Robert Koch Institute; pharmaceutical companies	http://www.influenza.rki.de/agi	A system for monitoring influenza in Germany, led by the Robert Koch Institute, Berlin, with German Green Cross, Marburg, and the National Reference Center for Influenza, Berlin	Open
144 Germany GENARS (German Network for Antimicrobial Resistance Surveillance)	Government of Germany/Federal Ministry of Health	http://www.genars.de/	The project is concerned with the collection and evaluation of antimicrobial resistance epidemiological data from microbiological institutes of German university clinics.	Open
145 Robert Koch Institute	Government of Germany/Federal Ministry of Health	http://www.rki.de/cln_011/nn_231704/EN/Content/Prevention/prevention__node__en.html__nnn=true	The tasks of the Robert Koch Institute include the monitoring of emerging diseases and risk factors in the general population, as well as the provision of scientific research.	Open
146 Salmonella Data Bank (SDB)	Government of Germany/Frankfurt an der Oder–Municipal Medical Investigation Office	Frankfurt an der Oder, Germany; URL not available	Creates a single salmonella reporting system that combines case reports, laboratory data, veterinary data, agricultural data, and labor statistics	Authorization
147 Indian Council of Medical Research (ICMR)	Government of India	http://www.icmr.nic.in/	Research priorities coincide with national health priorities, e.g., control and management of communicable diseases, etc.; searchable email and telephone directory; ICMR also has a list of medical research centers in India	Open

Table C.1—Continued

	Name	Sponsor	Location	Brief Description	Access
148	Ministry of Health, India	Government of India	http://www.mohfw.nic.in/depth.htm	Ministry of health Web site containing information for the general public and preparedness information for health professionals	Open
149	Central Bureau of Health Intelligence (CBHI)	Government of India/C3HI	http://cbhidghs.nic.in/	Provides ready information on various health indicators for India that are of great significance to the planners, policymakers, health administrators, research workers, and others engaged in raising the health and socioeconomic status of the country	Open
150	EPIFAR	Government of Italy/National Health Service (NHS)	http://www.ncbi.nlm.nih.gov/books/bv.fcgi?rid=hstat1.table.79221	Tracks individual prescription histories in order to provide estimates of disease prevalence	Open
151	Ministry of Health Jamaica	Government of Jamaica	http://www.moh.gov.jm/	Ministry of health Web site containing information for the general public and preparedness information for health professionals	Open
152	Ministry of Health, Japan	Government of Japan	http://www.mhlw.go.jp/english	Ministry of health Web site containing information for the general public and preparedness information for health professionals	Open
153	Infectious Disease Surveillance Center	Government of Japan/Ministry of Health, Labor and Welfare	http://idsc.nih.go.jp/	The infectious Disease Surveillance Center was established in 1997, replacing the Division of Infectious Disease Epidemiology.	Open
154	National Veterinary Assay Laboratory (NVAL)–Japanese Veterinary Antimicrobial Resistance Monitoring (JVARM)	Government of Japan/Ministry of Agriculture, Forestry and Fisheries	http://www.nval.go.jp/taisei/etaisei/JVARM(text%20and%20Fig)%20Final.htm	Web page with information and contact details for (JVARM)	Open
155	Ministry of Health, Lebanon	Government of Lebanon	http://www.public-health.gov.lb/index.shtml	Ministry of health Web site containing information for the general public and preparedness information for health professionals	Open
156	Ministry of Health Malaysia	Government of Malaysia	http://dph.gov.my/ddc/index.html	Ministry of health Web site containing information for the general public and preparedness information for health professionals	Open

Table C.1—Continued

Name	Sponsor	Location	Brief Description	Access
157 Border Infectious Disease Surveillance (BIDS) Project	Government of Mexico/Secretariat of Health; PAHO, HHS/ CDC; multiple U.S. and Mexican state health departments	http://www.azdhs.gov/phs/ borderhealth/bids.htm	Detects infectious disease along the U.S.-Mexico border	Authorization
158 Netherlands National Institute of Public Health and the Environment (RIVM) Surveillance System	Government of the Netherlands/ RIVM	http://www.epiet.org/ institutes/Bilthoven2004.htm	Catalogs and tracks resistance patterns of clinically isolated bacteria in the Netherlands	Within network
159 Ministry of Health, New Zealand	Government of New Zealand	http://www.moh.govt.nz/moh. nsf	Ministry of health Web site containing information for the general public and preparedness information for health professionals	Open
160 Disease Early Warning System (DEWS)	Government of Pakistan/National Institute of Health	http://www.gisdevelopment. net/magazine/gisdev/2003/ may/dewsi.shtml	Detects and predicts outbreaks and epidemics in Pakistan	Open
161 Ministry of Health, Saudi Arabia	Government of Saudi Arabia	http://www.moh.gov.sa/	Ministry of health Web site containing information for the general public and preparedness information for health professionals	Open
162 Ministry of Health, Singapore	Government of Singapore	http://www.moh.gov.sg/corp/ index.do	Ministry of health Web site containing information for the general public and preparedness information for health professionals	Open
163 Thailand National Antimicrobial Resistance Surveillance Center (NARST)	Government of Thailand/National Institute of Health	http://narst.dmsc.moph.go.th	Provides trend information based on research at the facility on antimicrobial drug resistance in Thailand for a variety of infectious organisms	Open
164 Uganda Disease Surveillance	Government of Uganda	http:// www.health.go.ug/ disease.htm	Cholera, HIV/AIDS, malaria, fever, and other transmittable diseases are continuously monitored to ensure that the area of infection in confined	Open
165 Communicable Disease Report Weekly, Health Protection Agency UK	Government of the UK/Health Protection Agency	http://www.hpa.org.uk/cdr/ default.htm	National public health bulletin for England and Wales	Open

Table C.1—Continued

Name	Sponsor	Location	Brief Description	Access
166 Public Health Laboratory Service (PHLS) Communicable Disease Surveillance Centre (CDSC)	Government of the UK/Health Protection Agency	http://www.hpa.org.uk/ infections/about/about.htm	Provides control, surveillance, and expert advice on the control of infectious disease	Open
167 UK Zoonotic Disease Surveillance	Government of the UK/Environment, Food, and Rural Affairs	http://www.noah.co.uk/ papers/defra_ab_resist_ surveillance_strat_0504.pdf	Strategy for the study of antimicrobial resistance trends among animals in England and Wales	Open
168 U.K. Food Micromodel (or Microbase)	Government of the UK/Food Standards Agency	http://www.food.gov. uk/science/research/ researchinfo/foodborneillness/ microriskresearch/ b12programme/B12projlist/	Allows the prediction of organism responses under a variety of conditions/stresses applied to food	Authorization
169 EpiMAN-FMD (foot-and-mouth disease) and EpiMAN-SF (swine fever)	Massey University, New Zealand; New Zealand Ministry of Agriculture	http://www.farmpro.co.nz/ devel-massey.asp	Assists disease-control authorities in the containment and eradication of animal disease outbreaks	Authorization
170 Regional Influenza Surveillance Group (GROG)	Northern France Reference Centre	http://www.grog.org/	Surveillance on the arrival and circulation of influenza viruses in France	Open
171 Scotland antimicrobial resistance information	Health Protection Scotland	http:// www.show.scot.nhs. uk/scieh/infectious/hai/SSHAIP/ antimicrobial_resistance.htm	Gateway site for antimicrobial resistance research in Scotland, including the Scottish Antimicrobial Resistance Surveillance program	Open
172 UK prion/Creutzfeldt-Jakob disease surveillance		http://www.cjd.ed.ac.uk/ PROTOCOL.htm	The incidence of CJD is monitored in the UK by the National CJD surveillance unit based at the Western General Hospital in Edinburgh, Scotland.	Open
Nongovernmental Organizations				
173 Biblio Directory for Infectious Disease	Geneva Foundation for Medical Education and Research, Geneva	http://www.gfmer.ch/ Medical_journals/Infectious_ diseases_microbiology_ tropical_medicine.htm	A database of links to medical journals for Infectious diseases, microbiology, tropical medicine	Open

Table C.1—Continued

Name	Sponsor	Location	Brief Description	Access
174 British Society for Antimicrobial Chemotherapy (BSAC) Resistance Surveillance Project	BSAC	http://www.bsacsurv.org/	The BSAC Resistance Surveillance Project monitors antimicrobial resistance in England, Wales, Scotland, Northern Ireland, and Ireland.	Open
175 Global Disaster Information Network (GDIN)	Global Disaster Information Network (GDIN)	http://www.gdin.org/wgl disease.html	An informational site on disasters (especially natural and chemical), providing maps, reports, press releases, and other information	Open
176 Rapid Emergency Digital Data Information Network (ReddiNet)	Hospital Association of Southern California	http://www.reddinet.com/	A communication network linking hospitals, emergency medical services agencies, first responders, and public health officials	Authorization
177 Russia Antibiotics ROSNET	Interregional Association for Clinical Microbiology and Antimicrobial Chemotherapy (IACMAC), Russia	http://www.iacmac.ru/iacmac/en/rosnet/	Russia's national network for monitoring of antibiotic resistance of both community-acquired and nosocomial infections	Open
178 National Foundation for Infectious Diseases (NFID)	NFID	http://www.nfid.org/	A nonprofit organization founded in 1973 that educates the public and healthcare professionals about the causes, treatment, and prevention of infectious diseases	Open
179 Infectious Disease Research Network	Various	http://www.idrn.org/	Network for research-sharing and collaboration with respect to infectious disease	Open
Professional/Academic				
180 Agriculture Network Information Center (AgNIC): Disease Announcements	Academic alliance	http://www.agnic.org/agnic/pmp	Searchable archive of the emerging plant disease announcements posted to the ProMED-mail mailing list	Open
181 American Veterinary Medical Association (AVMA)	AVMA	http://www.avma.org/disaster/default.asp	AVMA disaster preparedness guides	Open

Table C.1—Continued

Name	Sponsor	Location	Brief Description	Access
182 National Retail Data Monitor (NRDM)	Center for Biomedical Informatics, University of Pittsburgh	http://rods.health.pitt.edu/NRDM.htm	Monitors sales of over-the-counter health care products to identify disease outbreaks as early as possible; in operation since December 2002, there are nearly 20,000 retail pharmacy, grocery, and mass-merchandise stores that participate in the NRDM and more than 500 public health officials across 46 states, the District of Columbia, Puerto Rico, and the CDC have user accounts	Authorization
183 Centro de Investigaciones de Virosis Hemorrágicas y Enfermedades Transmisibles (CIVIHET)	CIVIHET	http://www.virus-venezuela.org/instituciones-centros.htm	A center of reference for dengue and viral hemorrhagic disease control in Venezuela (site is in Spanish)	Open
184 Biomedical Security Institute (BMSI)	Carnegie Mellon University; University of Pittsburgh	http://www.umc.pitt.edu/media/pcc001030/biomedical.html	The institute provides a preparedness detection and response capability network that can be used to rapidly and accurately respond to acts of bioterrorism	Authorization
185 Minnesota Microbiology Information System	Departments of Laboratory Medicine and Pathology and Medicine, University of Minnesota, Minneapolis	Departments of Laboratory Medicine and Pathology and Medicine University of Minnesota, Minneapolis; URL not available	This system provides Web-based access to inpatient microbiology results to reduce errors in data retrieval.	Authorization
186 Stepwise and Interactive Evaluation of Food Safety by an Expert System (SIEFE)	Dept. of Food Technology and Nutritional Sciences, Wageningen Agricultural University, the Netherlands	http://www.google.com/search?hl=en&q=Stepwise+and+Interactive+Evaluation+of+Food+safety+by+an+Expert+System+%28SIEFE%29 (information search)	Decision-support tool, provides microbiologic quantitative risk assessment for food products and their production processes	Open
187 European Committee on Antimicrobial Sensitivity Testing (EUCAST)	European Society of Clinical Microbiology and Infectious Disease	http://www.eucast.org/	Gateway site to the EUCAST system for monitoring antimicrobial resistance	Open

Table C.1—Continued

Name	Sponsor	Location	Brief Description	Access
188 FAS Terrorism Analysis	FAS	http:// www.fas.org/ahead/agroterror.htm	Analysis of methods to use disease surveillance to prepare for bioterrorism aimed at US agricultural systems. Also links to other FAS information, projects.	Open
189 Infectious Diseases Society of America (IDSA)	IDSA	http:// www.idsociety.org/	Professional association Web site, gateway for detailed information on infectious disease topics	Subscription
190 ProMed Mail searchable database	IDSA	http://www.promedmail.org/pls/promed/f?p=2400:1200:164551285136137I015	Searchable database of global disease outbreaks dedicated to the rapid dissemination of information on infectious diseases and acute exposures to toxins that affect human health, including those in animals and in plants grown for food or animal feed	Open
191 IDSA Emerging Infections Network (EIN)	Infectious Disease Society of America	http://www.idsociety.org/	Provider-based emerging infections sentinel network providing a resource for case detection and identification for health professionals	Subscription
192 ProMed Mail Daily update	Infectious Disease Society of America	http://www.promedmail.org/pls/askus/f?p=2400:1000:424240	Early warning system for emerging infectious diseases and toxins, including agroterrorism	Open
193 Microbiology Reference/ Resistance Surveillance	Mount Sinai Hospital; Toronto; Pfizer, Inc.	http://microbiology.mtsinai.on.ca/research/cbsn/default.asp	Surveillance of antimicrobial resistance at the Mount Sinai Hospital, Toronto, as part of the Canadian Bacterial Surveillance Network	Open
194 Virology Down Under, List of Diseases	Queensland University/Emerging Virus Group	http://www.uq.edu.au/vdu/InfectiousDiseaselinks.htm	A suite of pages providing information about a variety of human viruses, including RNA viruses and DNA viruses	Open
195 Intensive Care Antimicrobial Resistance Epidemiology ICARE	Rollins School of Public Health, Emory University; Abbott; AstraZeneca; bioMerieux; Elan; Pfizer, Inc.	http://www.sph.emory.edu/ICARE/index.php	Tracks antimicrobial resistance among pathogens responsible for nosocomial infections in ICUs	Open
196 Haemsept	Royal Victoria Hospital, Belfast, Northern Ireland	http://www.ncbi.nlm.nih.gov/books/bv.fcgi?rid=hstat1.table.79218	Detects bloodborne infections among hospitalized patients and provides guidance for antibiotic prescribing on a hematology unit	Authorization

Table C.1—Continued

Name	Sponsor	Location	Brief Description	Access
197 UK-Scotland Animal Disease Surveillance	Scottish Agricultural College	http://www.sac.ac.uk/ research/animalhealth/ researchteams/epidemiology/	Animal health epidemiology site in Scotland, UK	Open
198 Sociedad Venezolana de Infectologia (Infectious Diseases Society of Venenuela)	Sociedad Venezolana de Infectologia	http://www.svinfectologia. org/	This society deals with infectious diseases and antimicrobial resistance in Venezuela. Pathogens for antimicrobial resistance reporting Acinetobacter spp, Enterobacter cloacae, Enterococcus spp, E. coli, Haemophilus influenzae, Klebsiella spp, Neisseria meningitidis	Open
199 Bio-Spatio-Temporal Outbreak Reasoning Module (BioSTORM)	Stanford Medical Informatics, Stanford University	http://smi-web.stanford.edu/ projects/biostorm/research. htm	A research program to develop and evaluate intelligent systems for epidemic detection and characterization	Open
200 Computer-Assisted Infection (CAI) Monitoring Program	University Hospital of Tubingen, Germany	http://www.ncbi.nlm.nih. gov/books/bv.fcgi?rid=hstat1. table.79218	Integrates patient, lab, and epidemiologic surveillance of antibiotic-resistance data in order to manage nosocomial infections in ICU patients	Subscription
203 Rodent Disease Surveillance Program	University of Indiana (Urbana-Champaign)	http://www.dar.uiuc.edu/ disease.htm	Various fact sheets prepared on rodent diseases and surveillance of such diseases	Open
201 University of Alabama Data Mining Surveillance System (DMSS)	University of Alabama	http://www.medmined.com/ images/pdf/MIMPaper.pdf	Paper describing data-mining approaches for nosocomial infection surveillance; automatically identifies new, unexpected, and interesting patterns in surveillance data for infections that are not constrained to outbreaks for user-defined outcomes	Open
202 Knowledge-Based Information Network (WING) Giessen	University of Giessen, Germany	http://www.ncbi.nlm.nih. gov/books/bv.fcgi?rid=hstat1. table.79218	Detects nosocomial infections, even when only limited amounts of clinical data are available	Authorization
204 Realtime Outbreak and Disease Surveillance (RODS)	University of Pittsburgh; Carnegie Mellon University	http://rods.health.pitt.edu/	Open-source public health surveillance software, RODS collects and analyzes disease surveillance data in real time and has been in development since 1999 by the RODS laboratory	Authorization

Table C.1—Continued

Name	Sponsor	Location	Brief Description	Access
205 The Disaster Database Project	University of Richmond Dept of Emergency Services Mgmt.	http://cygnet.richmond.edu/is/esm/disaster/default.asp	Searchable database of disasters, including animal epidemics, epidemics, foodborne illness, mass outbreak, waterborne illness, occupational, and unknown afflictions	Open
206 Asian Network for Surveillance of Resistant Pathogens (ANSORP)	Various (primary: Samsung Medical Center, Sungkyunkwan University, Seoul, Korea)	http://www.ansorp.org/	Large collaborative study group for the antimicrobial resistance research in Asian countries	Open
207 GermWatcher	Washington University, St. Louis	http://www.computer.privateweb.at/judith/special_field3.htm#germwatcher	Nosocomial infection surveillance in Washington University (St. Louis, Mo.) hospitals, based on laboratory reports; detects outbreaks of new infections and rising endemic rates of preexisting infections	Authorization
208 World Veterinary Association (WVA)	WVA	http://www.worldvet.org/	Gateway site to information of interest to professional veterinarians worldwide	Open
Commercial				
209 Pig Disease Surveillance	5M Enterprises, Ltd.	http://www.thepigsite.com	Gateway site to all information related to pig farming and pork consumption	Open
210 Meteorological Information and Dispersion Assessment System Anti-Terrorism (MIDAS-AT)	ABS Consulting	http://www.absconsulting.com/midas/	Models attacks involving weapons of mass destruction using real-time meteorological data	Subscription
211 Animal Disease Surveillance Book	Blackwell Publishing	http:// www.vetsite.net/~cgilib/vetbook.asp?File=10022256	Directory of publications on a wide range of veterinary health issues, including abstract and information for the book Animal Disease Surveillance and Survey Systems	Open
212 Nuclear-Biological-Chemical Analysis	Bruhn-Newtech, UK/ Denmark	http://www.bnl-cbrn.co.uk/	Serves as a tool for risk management in emergency and training incidents involving hazardous materials	Subscription

Table C.1—Continued

Name	Sponsor	Location	Brief Description	Access
213 DOR BioPharma, Inc.	DOR BioPharma, Inc.	http://www.dorbiopharma.com/	Products in development are bioengineered vaccines designed to protect against the deadly effects of ricin and botulinum toxins, both of which are considered serious bioterrorism threats.	Authorization
214 Automated Decision Aid System for Hazardous Incidents (ADASHI)	Edgewood Chemical Biological Center	http://www.adashi.org/	Improves the response of military and civilian personnel to a biological or chemical incident; includes hazardous agent identification, source analysis, physical protection of responders, decontamination, medical treatment, casualty care, resources, and equipment	Subscription
215 Emergent Biosolutions	Emergent Biosolutions	http://www.emergentbiosolutions.com/home.asp	A biologics company focused on the research, development, and manufacture of vaccines and related products for prophylactic and therapeutic use against common diseases and biological weapons of mass destruction	Authorization
216 Epocrates Rx®/EpocratesID®	Epocrates, Inc.	http://www2.epocrates.com/products/rxpro/	A drug information program for use on handheld devices by clinicians	Subscription
217 Geographic Information System (GIS) Disease Surveillance	ESRI (Environmental Systems Research Institute, Inc.)	http://www.esri.com/industries/health/index.html	Product page for ESRI's ArcGIS mapping software in the health services field	Open
218 FirstWatch International chemical, biological, and nuclear (CBRN) data collection	First Watch International	http://www.firstwatchint.org/projects.html#nlr	Pay-for-use open-source intelligence service that uses a "software agent" to collect information on CBRN	Subscription
219 The Surveillance Network® (TSN®)	Focus Technologies USA	http://www.focustechnologies.com/bioinova/cms/cms.asp?cms_XIKI3320G	"World's largest electronic laboratory surveillance network and antimicrobial [resistance] profiling database"	Subscription
220 Chemical/Biological Operational Decision Aid (CODA)	General Dynamics Advanced Information Systems	http://www.veridian.com/offerings/suboffering.asp?offeringID=266&historyIDs=0,70,266	For the prediction of casualty and human performance-degradation analysis for military operations in the chemical, biological, and radiological environment	Subscription

Table C.1—Continued

Name	Sponsor	Location	Brief Description	Access
221 Global Expeditionary Medical System	Gerald Technologies, Inc. (contract DoD-USAF)	http://equalnox.com/eqnx/gems.shtml	Provides an integrated biohazard surveillance and detection system to keep a global watch over U.S. military forces	Subscription
222 Global Infectious Disease and Epidemiology Online Network (GIDEON)	GIDEON Informatics, Inc.	http://www.gideononline.com/	Web-based diagnostic tool of global infectious diseases and disease treatments	Subscription
223 GIS methods	GIS Development Pvt. Ltd.	http://www.gisdevelopment.net/application/health/links/ma0402abs.htm	Portal to GIS methods for surveillance purposes	Open
224 Biothreat Active Surveillance Integrated Information and Communication System (BASIICS)	Health Hero Network Inc.	http://www.pdacortex.com/BASIICS.htm	A pilot program for use the "Health Buddy" notifier device to transmit patient syndromic data to a local health authority	Authorization
225 Medcast	Healtheon Corp. and WebMD	http://www.webmd.com/	A commercial information service for practicing physicians; five nights a week, current medical news stories are summarized and formatted for delivery to the physician's office [Service may now be part of regular WebMD offerings]	Subscription
226 EMSystem™	Infinity Healthcare, Milwaukee	300 hospitals in 18 metropolitan regions in the United States and Melbourne, Australia; URL not available	EMSystem software is an Internet-based tool that can help manage hospital diversion status and collect real-time information for current and future planning by EMS agencies.	Subscription
227 Nuclear-biological-chemical command and control	Litton Integrated Systems (now part of Northrop Grumman)	URL not available	Provides decision-support during nuclear, biological, and chemical weapons events	Subscription
228 Antimicrobials, General Information	Medscape® (WebMD)	http://www.medscape.com/infectiousdiseaseshome	Gateway site to information contained in the Medscape online archives	Subscription
229 Motorola Emergency Medical Communications System	Motorola Corp.	URL not available	A wide-area radio communications network designed to enhance the delivery of emergency medical assistance to the public	Subscription

Table C.1—Continued

Name	Sponsor	Location	Brief Description	Access
230 Systematic Approach for Emergency Response (SAFER) Real-Time System	SAFER Corp.	http://www.safersystem.com/	Models toxic releases using real-time weather information	Subscription
231 Travax® EnCompass	Shoreland	http://shoreland.com/	Travax functions as a reference tool for travelers and traveling clinics. It provides country-specific information on diseases, immunizations, travel advisories, and WHO and CDC statements.	Subscription
232 SENTRY (Jones Group/ JMI Laboratories)	SmithKline Glaxo	http://www.fda.gov/ohrms/dockets/ac/03/slides/3919S2_03_Carnevale/sld030.htm	A longitudinal surveillance program designed to track antimicrobial resistance patterns of nosocomial and community-acquired infections	Open
233 The Economist: Economist Intelligence Unit	The Economist	http://www.eiu.com/	Risk assessments for over 200 separate countries that include reporting of violent incidents	Subscription
234 National Flu Surveillance Network (NFSN)	ZymeTx, Inc.	http://www.fluwatch.com/	Produces virtual real-time reports to keep the public and public health officials alerted to the movement of flu across the United States	Open

NOTE: All information listed in the table is current as of the period during which data were collected for this study, July through October 2005. Some descriptions in the table are included as self-reported by the individual sources.

References

Albright, Penrose C., Assistant Under Secretary for Science and Technology, U.S. Department of Homeland Security, testimony before the Senate Committee on Health, Education, Labor, and Pensions, February 8, 2005.

APEC—*see* Asia-Pacific Economic Cooperation.

Armstrong, Gregory L., Laura A. Conn, and Robert W. Pinner, "Trends in Infectious Disease Mortality in the United States During the 20th Century," *Journal of the American Medical Association*, Vol. 281, No. 1, January 6, 1999, pp. 61–66.

Asia-Pacific Economic Cooperation, APEC Initiative to Strengthen Health Security, 2003/AMM/024, Agenda Item V.6, 15th APEC Ministerial Meeting, Bangkok, October 17–18, 2003.

Berlinguer, Giovanni, "The Interchange of Disease and Health Between the Old and New Worlds," *American Journal of Public Health*, Vol. 82, No. 10, October 1992, pp. 1407–1413.

———, "Bioethics, Human Security, and Global Health," in Lincoln Chen, Jennifer Leaning, and Vasant Narasimhan, eds., *Global Health Challenges for Human Security*, Cambridge, Mass.: Harvard University Press, 2003, pp. 53–65.

Bettcher, D., and K. Lee, "Globalisation and Public Health," *Journal of Epidemiology and Community Health*, Vol. 56, No. 1, January 2002, pp. 8–17.

Brower, Jennifer, and Peter Chalk, *The Global Threat of New and Reemerging Infectious Diseases: Reconciling U.S. National Security and Public Health Policy*, Santa Monica, Calif.: RAND Corporation, MR-1602-RC, 2003. Online at http://www.rand.org/pubs/monograph_reports/MR1602/index.html (as of June 12, 2006).

Caldwell, Blake, "Biosense: Using Health Data for Early Event Detection and Situational Awareness," briefing, February 23, 2006. Online at http://dimacs.rutgers.edu/Workshops/Surveillance/slides/caldwell.ppt (as of May 2, 2006).

Cash, Richard A., and Vasant Narasimhan, "Impediments to Global Surveillance of Infectious Diseases: Consequences of Open Reporting in a Global Economy," *Bulletin of the World Health Organization*, Vol. 78, No. 11, 2000, pp. 1358–1367. Online at http://whqlibdoc.who.int/bulletin/2000/Number%2011/78(11)1358-1367.pdf (as of June 12, 2006).

CDC—see Centers for Disease Control and Prevention.

Center for Strategic International Studies, *Contagion and Conflict: Health as a Global Security Challenge*, Washington, D.C., 2000.

Centers for Disease Control and Prevention, *Addressing Emerging Infectious Disease Threats: A Prevention Strategy for the United States*, Atlanta, Ga.: National Center for Infectious Diseases, Centers for Disease Control and Prevention, U.S. Department of Health and Human Services, 1994. Online at ftp://ftp.cdc.gov/pub/infectious_diseases/emergplan/pdf/emergplan.pdf (as of June 12, 2006).

————, *Preventing Emerging Infectious Diseases: A Strategy for the 21st Century*, Atlanta, Ga.: National Center for Infectious Diseases, Centers for Disease Control and Prevention, U.S. Department of Health and Human Services, October, 1998. Online at http://www.cdc.gov/ncidod/emergplan/plan98.pdf (as of June 12, 2006).

Chen, Lincoln, and Vasant Narasimhan, "A Human Security Agenda for Global Health," in Lincoln Chen, Jennifer Leaning, and Vasant Narasimhan, eds., *Global Health Challenges for Human Security*, Cambridge, Mass.: Harvard University Press, 2003, pp. 3–12.

Chyba, Christopher F., *Biological Terrorism, Emerging Diseases, and National Security*, New York: Rockefeller Brothers Fund Project on World Security, 1998.

CISET—*see* Committee on International Science, Engineering, and Technology.

Cohen, Mitchell L., "Changing Patterns of Infectious Disease," *Nature*, Vol. 406, No. 6797, August 17, 2000, pp. 762–767.

Commission on Human Security, *Final Report of the Commission on Human Security*, New York, May 1, 2003. Online at http://www.humansecurity-chs.org/finalreport/index.html (as of October 8, 2005).

Committee on International Science, Engineering, and Technology, *Infectious Diseases: A Global Health Threat*, Washington, D.C.: U.S. National Science and Technology Council Committee on International Science, Engineering, and Technology (CISET) Working Group on Emerging and Re-Emerging Infectious Diseases, 1995.

Crosse, Marcia, *Influenze Pandemic: Challenges in Preparedness and Response*, testimony before the House Committee on Government Reform, Washington, D.C.: U.S. Government Accountability Office, GAO-05-863T, June 30, 2005. Online at http://www.gao.gov/new.items/d05863t.pdf (as of June 12, 2006).

Elbe, Stefan, "HIV/AIDS and the Changing Landscape of War in Africa," *International Security*, Vol. 27, No. 2, Fall 2002, pp. 159–177.

Enemark, Christian, *Disease Security in Northeast Asia: Biological Weapons and Natural Plagues*, Canberra: Strategic and Defence Studies Centre, The Australian National University, 2004.

Evans, Graham, and Jeffrey Newnham, *The Dictionary of World Politics: A Reference Guide to Concepts, Ideas and Institutions*, London: Harvester Wheatsheaf, 1992. Cited in Kelley Lee, Kent Buse, and Suzanne Fustukian, eds., *Health Policy in a Globalising World*, London: Cambridge University Press, 2002.

Fidler, David P., "Return of the Fourth Horseman: Emerging Infectious Diseases and International Law," *Minnesota Law Review*, Vol. 81, No. 4, April 1997, pp. 771–868.

Fidler, David P., David L. Heyman, S. M. Ostroff, and Thomas F. O'Brien, "Emerging and Reemerging Infectious Diseases: Challenges for International, National, and State Law," *International Lawyer*, Vol. 31, No. 3, 1997, pp. 773–800.

Fields, Gary, "Suspicious Cargo: For U.S. Customs, Trade and Security Clash on the Docks—War on Terror Has Inspectors Examining More Ships, Delaying More Deliveries—Opening 1,600 Bags of Cumin," *Wall Street Journal*, September 12, 2002, pp. 1–2.

Flanagan, Stephen J., Ellen L. Frost, and Richard L. Kugler, *Challenges of the Global Century: Report of the Project on Globalization and National Security*, Washington, D.C.: Institute for National Strategic Studies, National Defense University, June 2001. Online at http://www.ndu.edu/inss/books/ Books_2001/Challenges%20of%20the%20Global%20Century%20June%202001/CHALENG. PDF (as of June 12, 2006).

Frist, Bill, "The Threat of Avian Flu: U.S. Needs an Action Plan—and Needs It Now," editorial, *Washington Times*, September 29, 2005.

Gabriel, Richard A., and Karen S. Metz, *A History of Military Medicine*, 2 vols., New York: Greenwood Publishing Group, 1992.

Garrett, Laurie, "The Next Pandemic?" *Foreign Affairs*, Vol. 84, No. 4, July/August 2005. Online at http://www.foreignaffairs.org/20050701faessay84401/laurie-garrett/the-next-pandemic.html (as of June 12, 2006).

Gottron, Frank, *Project Bioshield*, Washington, D.C.: Congressional Research Service, RS21507, July 23, 2003.

Heymann, David L., "Evolving Infectious Disease Threats to National and Global Security," in Lincoln Chen, Jennifer Leaning, and Vasant Narasimhan, eds., *Global Health Challenges for Human Security*, Cambridge, Mass.: Harvard University Press, 2003, pp. 105–123.

Heymann, David L., and Guénaël R. Rodier, "Global Surveillance of Communicable Diseases," *Emerging Infectious Diseases*, Vol. 4, No. 3, July–September 1998, pp. 362–265. Online at http:// www.cdc.gov/ncidod/eid/vol4no3/heymann.htm (as of June 12, 2006).

Howson, Christopher P., Harvey V. Fineberg, and Barry R. Bloom, "The Pursuit of Global Health: The Relevance of Engagement for Developed Countries," *The Lancet*, Vol. 351, No. 9102, February 21, 1998, pp. 586–590.

Huang, Yanzhong, *Mortal Peril: Public Health in China and Its National Security Implications*, Washington, D.C.: Chemical and Biological Arms Control Institute, Health and Security Series Special Report 7, 2003.

Institute of Medicine, *America's Vital Interest in Global Health: Protecting Our People, Enhancing Our Economy, and Advancing Our International Interests*, Washington, D.C.: National Academy Press, 1997.

Johnson, Niall P. A. S, and Juergen Mueller, "Updating the Accounts: Global Mortality of the 1918– 1920 'Spanish' Influenza Pandemic," *Bulletin of the History of Medicine*, Vol. 76, No. 1, Spring 2002, pp. 105–115.

Lederberg, Joshua S., "Infectious Disease as an Evolutionary Paradigm," *Emerging Infectious Diseases*, Vol. 3, No. 4, October–December 1997, pp. 417–423. Online at http://www.cdc.gov/ncidod/eid/ vol3no4/lederber.htm (as of June 12, 2006).

Lederberg, Joshua S., Robert E. Shope, and Stanley C. Oaks, Jr., eds., *Emerging Infections: Microbial Threats to Health in the United States*, Washington, D.C.: National Academy Press, 1992.

Lee, Kelley, Kent Buse, and Suzanne Fustukian, eds., *Health Policy in a Globalising World*, London: Cambridge University Press, 2002.

Levy, Craig E., and Kenneth L. Gage, "Plague in the United States, 1995–1997," *Infections in Medicine*, Vol. 16, No. 1, 1999, pp. 54–64.

Lounibos, L. Philip, "Invasions by Insect Vectors of Human Disease," *Annual Review of Entomology*, Vol. 47, January 2002, pp. 233–266.

Martinez-Lopez, Lester, Commanding General, U.S. Army Medical Research and Materiel Command, testimony before the House Committee on Veterans' Affairs, August 26, 2004.

McKibbin, Warwick J., and Alexandra A. Sidorenko, "Global Macroeconomic Consequences of Pandemic Influenza," Lowy Institute for International Policy, Australian Centre for Economic Research on Health, February 2006. Online at http://www.lowyinstitute.org/Publication.asp?pid=345 (as of June 12, 2006).

McQueary, Charles E., Under Secretary for Science and Technology, U.S. Department of Homeland Security, testimony before the House Committee on Science, Washington, D.C., February 16, 2005.

Mills, Christina E., James M. Robins, and Marc Lipsitch, "Transmissibility of 1918 Pandemic Influenza," *Nature*, Vol. 432, No. 7019, December 16, 2004, pp. 904–906.

Moore, Chester G., and Carl J. Mitchell, "*Aedes albopictus* in the United States: Ten-Year Presence and Public Health Implications," *Emerging Infectious Diseases*, Vol. 3, No. 3, July–September 1997, pp. 329–334. Online at http://www.cdc.gov/ncidod/eid/vol3no3/moore.htm (as of June 12, 2006).

Moore, Melinda, Philip Gould, and Barbara S. Keary, "Global Urbanization and Impact on Health," *International Journal of Hygiene and Environmental Health*, Vol. 206, Nos. 4–5, August 2003, pp. 269–278.

Morr, Karen, Acting Assistant Secretary for Information Analysis, U.S. Department of Homeland Security, testimony before the House Subcommittee on Emergency Preparedness, Science and Technology, Washington, D.C., July 12, 2005.

National Center for Health Statistics, *Table LCWK 1: Deaths, Percent of Total Deaths, and Death Rates for the 15 Leading Causes of Death in 5-Year Age Groups, by Race and Sex: United States, 2000*, Hyattsville, Md.: U.S. Centers for Disease Control and Prevention, U.S. Department of Health and Human Services, 2000. Online at http://www.cdc.gov/nchs/data/dvs/LCWK1_2000.pdf (as of February 8, 2006).

Navarro, Vicente, "Comment: Whose Globalization?" *American Journal of Public Health*, Vol. 88, No. 5, May 1998, pp. 742–743.

O'Brien, Thomas F., "Emergence, Spread, and Environmental Effect of Antimicrobial Resistance: How Use of an Antimicrobial Anywhere Can Increase Resistance to Any Antimicrobial Anywhere Else," *Clinical Infectious Diseases*, Vol. 34, No. S3, June 1, 2002, pp. S78–S84. Online at http://www.journals.uchicago.edu/CID/journal/issues/v34nS3/020123/020123.web.pdf (as of June 12, 2006).

Office of Science and Technology Policy, *Science and Technology: A Foundation for Homeland Security*, Washington, D.C.: Executive Office of the President of the United States, April 2005. Online at http://www.ostp.gov/html/OSTPHomeland.pdf (as of June 12, 2006).

Ostergard, Robert L., Jr., "Politics in the Hot Zone: AIDS and National Security in Africa," *Third World Quarterly*, Vol. 23, No. 2, April 1, 2002, pp. 333–350.

Osterholm, Michael T., "Preparing for the Next Pandemic," *Foreign Affairs*, Vol. 84, No. 4, July/August 2005. Online at http://www.foreignaffairs.org/20050701faessay84402/michael-t-osterholm/preparing-for-the-next-pandemic.html (as of June 12, 2006).

Oxford, J. S., R. Lambkin, A. Sefton, R. Daniels, A. Elliot, R. Brown, and D. Gill, "A Hypothesis: The Conjunction of Soldiers, Gas, Pigs, Ducks, Geese and Horses in Northern France During the Great War Provided the Conditions for the Emergence of the 'Spanish' Influenza Pandemic of 1918–1919," *Vaccine*, Vol. 23, No. 7, January 4, 2005, pp. 940–945.

Pinner, R. W., S. M. Teutsch, L. Simonsen, L. A. Klug, J. M. Graber, M. J. Clarke, and R. L. Berkelman, "Trends in Infectious Diseases Mortality in the United States," *Journal of the American Medical Association*, Vol. 275, No. 3, January 17, 1996, pp. 189–193.

Pomfret, John, "China's Slow Reaction to Fast-Moving Illness," *Washington Post*, April 3, 2003, p. A18.

Price-Smith, A. T., *Pretoria's Shadow: The HIV/AIDS Pandemic and National Security in South Africa*, CBACI Health and Security Series, Special Report 4, Washington, D.C.: Chemical and Biological Arms Control Institute, 2002.

Public Law 107-188, Public Health Security and Bioterrorism Preparedness and Response Act, June 12, 2002.

Rodier, G. R., M. J. Ryan, and D. L. Heymann, "Global Epidemiology of Infectious Diseases," in G. T. Strickland, ed., *Hunter's Tropical Medicine and Emerging Infectious Diseases*, 8th ed., Philadelphia: W. B. Saunders Company, 2000.

Roemer, Milton I., "Comment: The Globalization of Public Health," *American Journal of Public Health*, Vol. 88, No. 5, May 1998, p. 744.

Rothschild, Emma, "What Is Security? (The Quest for World Order)," *Daedalus*, Vol. 124, No. 3, Summer 1995, pp. 53–98.

Shea, Dana A., *The National Biodefense Analysis and Countermeasures Center: Issues for Congress*, Washington, D.C.: Congressional Research Service, RL32891, April 25, 2005.

Shisana, Olive, Nompumelelo Zungu-Dirwayi, and William Shisana, "AIDS: A Threat to Human Security," in Lincoln Chen, Jennifer Leaning, and Vasant Narasimhan, eds., *Global Health Challenges for Human Security*, Cambridge, Mass.: Harvard University Press, 2003, pp. 141–160.

Smallman-Raynor, M. R., and A. D. Cliff, "Impact of Infectious Diseases on War," *Infectious Disease Clinics of North America*, Vol. 18, No. 2, 2004, pp. 341–368.

Smolinski, Mark S., Margaret A. Hamburg, and Joshua Lederberg, eds., *Microbial Threats to Health: Emergence, Detection, and Response*, Washington, D.C.: Board on Global Health, Institute of Medicine, National Academies Press, 2003.

Stewart, William H., "A Mandate for State Action," presented at the Association of State and Territorial Health Officers, Washington, D.C., December 4, 1967.

Store, Jonas Gahr, Jonathan Welch, and Lincoln Chen, "Health and Security for a Global Century," in Lincoln Chen, Jennifer Leaning, and Vasant Narasimhan, eds., *Global Health Challenges for Human Security*, Cambridge, Mass.: Harvard University Press, 2003, pp. 66–84.

Szreter, Simon, "Health and Security in Historical Perspective," in Lincoln Chen, Jennifer Leaning, and Vasant Narasimhan, eds., *Global Health Challenges for Human Security*, Cambridge, Mass.: Harvard University Press, 2003, pp. 31–52.

Trampuz, Andrej, Rajesh M. Prabhu, Thomas F. Smith, and Larry M. Baddour, "Avian Influenza: A New Pandemic Threat?" *Mayo Clinic Proceedings*, Vol. 79, No. 4, April 2004, pp. 523–530. Online at http://www.mayoclinicproceedings.com/pdf%2F7904%2F7904crc%2Epdf (as of June 12, 2006).

UNAIDS, *Report on the Global HIV/AIDS Epidemic*, Barcelona Report, CP065, Geneva: Joint UN Programme on HIV/AIDS, July 2002.

———, *2004 Report on the Global HIV/AIDS Epidemic: Executive Summary*, Geneva: Joint UN Programme on HIV/AIDS, June 2004. Online at http://www.unaids.org/bangkok2004/GAR2004_pdf/GAR2004_Execsumm_en.pdf (as of June 12, 2006).

United Nations, *United Nations Millennium Development Goals*, 2000. Online at http://www.un.org/millenniumgoals/ (as of October 5, 2005).

United Nations Development Programme, *Human Development Report 1994*, Oxford: Oxford University Press, 1994. Online at http://hdr.undp.org/reports/global/1994/en/ (as of June 12, 2006).

———, *Human Development Report 2005: International Cooperation at a Crossroads—Aid, Trade, and Security in an Unequal World*, New York, 2005. Online at http://hdr.undp.org/reports/global/2005/pdf/HDR05_complete.pdf (as of November 7, 2005).

United Nations Security Council, Security Council Resolution 1308 (2000) on the Responsibility of the Security Council in the Maintenance of International Peace and Security: HIV/AIDS and International Peacekeeping Operations, 4,172nd meeting, Geneva, July 17, 2000. Online at http://www.reliefweb.int/w/rwb.nsf/0/d1261fd7ea89821c85256b8000774bfb?OpenDocument (as of July 19, 2005).

U.S. Customs and Border Protection, "Fact Sheet: Trade," Washington, D.C., undated. Online at http://www.cbp.gov/linkhandler/cgov/newsroom/fact_sheets/press_kit/trade_press.ctt/trade_press.pdf (as of June 12, 2006).

U.S. Department of Energy, "Department of Homeland Security Under Secretary to Dedicate New Biodefense Knowledge Center," press release, Lawrence Livermore National Laboratory, Livermore, Calif., September 10, 2004.

U.S. Department of Health and Human Services, *HHS Pandemic Influenza Plan*, Washington, D.C., November 2005. Online at http://www.hhs.gov/pandemicflu/plan/pdf/HHSPandemicInfluenzaPlan.pdf (as of November 7, 2005).

U.S. Department of Homeland Security, *National Response Plan*, Washington, D.C., December 2004. Online at http://www.dhs.gov/interweb/assetlibrary/NRP_FullText.pdf (as of November 7, 2005).

———, "Fact Sheet: National Biodefense Analysis and Countermeasures Center," Washington, D.C., February 24, 2005. Online at http://www.dhs.gov/dhspublic/display?content=4377 (as of June 12, 2006).

U.S. Department of State, *U.S. International Strategy on HIV/AIDS*, publication number 10296, Washington, D.C., July 1995. Online at http://dosfan.lib.uic.edu/ERC/environment/releases/9507.html (as of October 1, 2005).

U.S. General Accounting Office, *Global Health: Framework for Infectious Disease Surveillance*, GAO/ NSIAD-00-205R, Washington, D.C., July 20, 2000a. Online at http://www.gao.gov/new.items/ ns00205r.pdf (as of June 12, 2006).

————, *West Nile Virus Outbreak: Lessons for Public Health Preparedness*, GAO/HEHS-00-180, Washington, D.C., September 2000b. Online at http://www.gao.gov/archive/2000/he00180.pdf (as of June 12, 2006).

————, *Global Health: Challenges in Improving Infectious Disease Surveillance Systems*, GAO-01-722, Washington, D.C., August 2001. Online at http://www.gao.gov/new.items/d01722.pdf (as of June 12, 2006).

U.S. Government Accountability Office, *Emerging Infectious Diseases: Asian SARS Outbreak Challenged International and National Responses*, GAO-04-564, Washington, D.C., April 2004. Online at http://www.gao.gov/new.items/d04564.pdf (as of June 12, 2006).

————, *Information Technology: Federal Agencies Face Challenges in Implementing Initiatives to Improve Public Health Infrastructure*, GAO-05-308, Washington, D.C., June 2005. Online at http://www. gao.gov/new.items/d05308.pdf (as of June 12, 2006).

U.S. National Intelligence Council, *National Intelligence Estimate: The Global Infectious Disease Threat and Its Implications for the United States*, Washington, D.C., NIE 99-17D, January 2000. Online at http://www.dni.gov/nic/PDF_GIF_otherprod/infectiousdisease/infectiousdiseases.pdf (as of June 12, 2006).

Vitko, John, Jr., Director, Biological Countermeasures Portfolio, Science and Technology Directorate, U.S. Department of Homeland Security, statement before the House Committee on Homeland Security, Subcommittee on Prevention of Nuclear and Biological Attack, Washington, D.C., July 28, 2005.

White House, "Fact Sheet: Addressing the Threat of Emerging Infectious Diseases," press release regarding Presidential Decision Directive NTSC-7, Washington, D.C.: Office of Science and Technology Policy, June 12, 1996a. Online at http://www.fas.org/irp/offdocs/pdd_ntsc7.htm (as of June 8, 2005).

————, "Vice President Announces Policy on Infectious Diseases: New Presidential Policy Calls for Coordinated Approach to Global Issue," Washington, D.C.: Office of the Vice President, June 12, 1996b. Online at http://www.fas.org/irp/offdocs/pdd_ntsc7.htm [second item] (as of June 8, 2005).

————, *The National Security Strategy of the United States of America*, Washington, D.C., September 2002. Online at http://www.whitehouse.gov/nsc/nss.pdf (as of June 12, 2006).

————, *Homeland Security Presidential Directive 10 and National Security Directive Presidential 33: Biodefense for the 21st Century*, Washington, D.C., April 28, 2004. Online at http://www.white house.gov/homeland/20040430.html (as of June 12, 2006).

————, *National Strategy for Pandemic Influenza*, Washington, D.C.: Homeland Security Council, November 2005. Online at http://www.whitehouse.gov/homeland/nspi.pdf (as of November 7, 2005).

Wilder-Smith, Annelies, Timothy M. S. Barkham, Arul Earnest, and Nicholas I. Paton, "Acquisition of W135 Meningococcal Carriage in Hajj Pilgrims and Transmission to House Contacts: Prospective Study," *British Medical Journal*, Vol. 325, No. 7360, August 17, 2002, pp. 365–366.

Wilson, Mary E., "The Power of Plague," *Epidemiology*, Vol. 6, No. 4, 1995a, pp. 458–460.

———, "Travel and the Emergence of Infectious Diseases," *Emerging Infectious Diseases*, Vol. 1, No. 2, April–June 1995b, pp. 39–46. Online at http://www.cdc.gov/ncidod/eid/vol1no2/wilson. htm (as of June 12, 2006).

———, "Health and Security: Globalization of Infectious Diseases," in Lincoln Chen, Jennifer Leaning, and Vasant Narasimhan, eds., *Global Health Challenges for Human Security*, Cambridge, Mass.: Harvard University Press, 2003a, pp. 87–104.

———, "The Traveler and Emerging Infections: Sentinel, Courier, Transmitter," *Journal of Applied Microbiology*, Vol. 94, No. S1, May 2003b, pp. 1–11.

Woolhouse, Mark E. J., and Chris Dye, eds., "Preface," introduction to theme issue, "Population Biology of Emerging and Reemerging Pathogens," *Philosophical Transactions of the Royal Society for Biological Sciences*, Vol. 356, No. 1411, July 29, 2001, pp. 981–982. Online at http://www.journals. royalsoc.ac.uk/media/n9mktvqqqp93k6wywq3m/contributions/q/y/0/l/qy0leb2h83mcgju4.pdf (as of June 12, 2006).

World Health Assembly, Communicable Disease Prevention and Control: New Emerging and Re-Emerging Infectious Diseases, Resolution 48.13, Geneva, May 12, 1995.

———, Revision of the International Health Regulations, Resolution 56.28, Geneva, May 28, 2003. Online at http://www.who.int/gb/ebwha/pdf_files/WHA56/ea56r28.pdf (as of June 12, 2006).

World Health Organization, *Declaration of Alma-Ata: International Conference on Primary Health Care, Alma-Ata, USSR, 6–12 September 1978*, Alma-Ata, USSR, 1978. Online at http://www.who. int/hpr/NPH/docs/declaration_almaata.pdf (as of October 25, 2005).

———, *The World Health Report 1996: Fighting Disease, Fostering Development*, Geneva, 1996. Online at http://www.who.int/whr/1996/en/ (as of September 8, 2005).

———, *Report of the WHO Commission on Macroeconomics and Health*, Geneva, April 23, 2002. Online at http://www.who.int/gb/ebwha/pdf_files/WHA55/ea555.pdf (as of October 25, 2005).

———, *Summary of Probable SARS Cases with Onset of Illness from 1 November to 31 July 2003*, Geneva, data as of December 31, 2003. Online at http://www.who.int/csr/sars/country/table2004_ 04_21/en/index.html (as of October 24, 2005).

———, *The World Health Report 2004: Changing History*, Geneva, 2004. Online at http://www.who. int/whr/2004/en/report04_en.pdf (as of October 19, 2005).

———, *International Health Regulations*, third report of Committee A, 58th World Health Assembly, Geneva, May 23, 2005. Online at http://www.who.int/gb/ebwha/pdf_files/WHA58/A58_55- en.pdf (as of September 8, 2005).

———, "Ten Things You Need to Know About Pandemic Influenza," Geneva, October 14, 2005b. Online at http://www.who.int/csr/disease/influenza/pandemic10things/en/ (as of April 26, 2006).

Yach, Derek, and Douglas Bettcher, "The Globalization of Public Health, I: Threats and Opportunities," *American Journal of Public Health*, Vol. 88, No. 5, May 1998a, pp. 735–737.

———, "The Globalization of Public Health, II: The Convergence of Self-Interest and Altruism," *American Journal of Public Health*, Vol. 88, No. 5, May 1998b, pp. 738–740.

Zacher, Mark W., "Global Surveillance of Communicable Diseases," in Inge Kaul, Isabelle Grunberg, and Marc A. Stern, eds., *Global Public Goods*, New York: Oxford University Press, 1999, pp. 266–284.